Macrobiotic
Home Food Processing

Macrobiotic Home Food Processing

By Guy Lalumiere

Foreword byAveline Kushi

with Illustrations
by the Author and Lily Kushi

Published by One Peaceful World Press, Becket, Massachusetts, U.S.A.

For information on mail-order sales, wholesale or retail discounts, distribution, translations, and foreign rights, please contact the publisher:

One Peaceful World Press
P.O. Box 10
Leland Road
Becket, MA 01223
U.S.A.

Telephone (413) 623-2322
Fax (413) 623-8827

First Edition: June 1993
10 9 8 7 6 5 4 3 2 1

ISBN 1-882984-00-5

Printed in the United States of America

Contents

Foreword

By Aveline Kushi

For the last forty years, my constant dream has been to introduce healthful and delicious traditional foods from all over the world to this country. Of course, I wanted to introduce tofu, miso, and shoyu from Japan, but also foods such as tempeh, which originated in Indonesia and which I discovered nearly twenty years ago in Holland!

Tempeh has now become a staple of the natural foods movement. Nearly fifteen years ago, in Venezuela, I was introduced to corn masa, or whole corn dough, another delightful food. (In Brookline Anna Troconis and Armando and Maritza Rojas taught traditional cooking with corn at the Kushi Institute.) On a visit to Europe, I discovered that tempura was native to Portugal and brought to Japan four hundred years ago. Noodles, of course, originated in China and were brought to Italy and became spaghetti. In this way, delicious, healthful foods from East and West have crisscrossed the world.

My wish has always been to encourage people to grow their own organic grains and vegetables, to respect the soil, and to be self-reliant. To me, the wonderful international exchange of foods and recipes, such as the home processing methods presented in this book, are a joyful way to realize our common goal of a healthy, peaceful world.

Guy Lalumiere's patience, dedication, and beautiful personality made him the perfect person to learn—and then teach—this age-old tradition. I remember when I recommended to him that he go to Japan to study and deepen his understanding. He went with such enthusiasm and dedication that, in a remarkably short time, he was able to master the technology and techniques of food processing and bring back his precious knowledge to the West. For several years now, he has been teaching and making these methods available. His skill is truly a blessing for everyone who has the opportunity to enjoy his delicious products. Wonderful sourdough bread, in particular, has gained Guy many admirers.

While he was studying miso-making in Japan, Japanese television correspondents interviewed him, and broadcast new stories of his daily life, eating brown rice, natto, and other simple foods and studying age-old hand methods of traditional food preparation. Thanks to Guy's influence, many Japanese began to reconsider their own traditions which are slowly disappearing from modern Japan. Such international exchange is priceless!

It has been my life-long belief that in the peace and tranquility of our kitchens, through the exchange of whole organic foods, recipes, and knowledge of home-processing techniques, we can heal and pacify our confused and chaotic society, respect our status as human beings, and preserve our planet and its beautiful natural environment.

The methods in this book have been passed down to us through countless generations. I am thankful to Guy for making them available to many readers. I am grateful to him for his dedication and willingness to share the knowledge and expertise which he has developed through years of patient work and study. His instructions are clear, easy to follow, and the results are so enjoyable. It is my hope that many of you reading this book will also try and enjoy making these delicious foods and passing them on to your children and grandchildren.

Becket, Massachusetts
March 23, 1993

Introduction

This book is about transmutation. It shows ways to completely change the nature of some very common foods. It describes
ways to create foods which have very unique properties, not
found in the ingredients they are made from.

In the distant past, some wise alchemists discovered
many surprising secrets of nature lying dormant beneath the
skins of our most common staple foods. Take soybeans, for
example. When cooked they make a very warming, hearty
dish. Transformed into tofu, their properties change completely: tofu is light and cool. Or take tamari and hatcho miso,
both made from soybeans. Their transformation gives products with a host of wonderful properties which soybeans
alone do not have. Their nature has been changed. Some kind
of transmutation has occurred.

Or take wheat berries, grind them into flour, add salt
and water. With these, you can make either bread or noodles.
Even though chemically, their compositon is very similar,
they are two completely different foods. And they are also
completely different from wheat berries cooked in water with
salt. Bread is heavy and very warming, good to eat when you
do physical work; noodles are light and cooling, just the right
food to do intellectual work. The transformation has changed
the nature of wheat, some kind of transmutation has also hap-
pened.

Say, for instance, you want a source of protein that is
light and cooling, as when it is hot outside, or when you do
little physical work. All meats are warming and heavy; beans
also. You might choose fish, but you would have to eat it raw,

as in sushi. But then, it would strongly activate you because you eat the vitality of the fish. Only tofu would satisfy. It has unique properties not found anywhere else.

The alchemists of the past discovered something very important. They taught their discoveries to the next generation which refined and developed the original processes. They, in turn, handed down to their apprentices the results of their work. Miso, bread, tofu, and many other foods have evolved this way for many centuries. They have come to us enriched with the experience and dedication of many generations. They have changed considerably over the centuries. But, still, they have remained essentially the same, always manifesting their magical properties whenever we ask for them.

The most common items, such as wheat, rice, or soybeans, can be transformed into hundreds of unique foods with the help of a few "magical" ingredients (salt, nigari, spores of certain molds, wood ashes, etc.), the right temperature, and, most important, the right time. Experienced cooks usually say that the most difficult foods to make are those that contain only one ingredient. With only one item, you cannot hide a defect, you cannot change one taste with another. The secrets of these foods lie in the right time, or we might say correct timing, and also right temperature, that is, the appropriate environment—moisture, climate, and season—for all fermented foods and the right amount of fire for all cooked foods.

These preparations have been made by many people for many centuries. When you first try making them, of course, you should not expect to accomplish a masterpiece right away. The secrets of these foods lie in the process itself. It is that part you should pursue, not the finished product. Forget about the philosopher's stone.

During the last century or so, the all important preparation of these foods has been left in the hands of scientists and engineers. They may be accomplished chemists (maybe excessively so), but many of them are very poor alchemists. This book has been written to awaken talents lying dormant in everyone, which are urgently needed today. It is also written with the hope that these foods, which have been handed down to us, will live safely through this century, and be carried on by the next generations.

I have been learning about these foods for many years. My studies brought me to Europe and Japan. I owe everything I know to all the people who have anonymously made these foods all their life. No one owns a copyright on bread or miso. I am indebted to Michio and Aveline Kushi for inspiring me on this journey.

I am not a writer. I would be incapable of "kneading" a book together, even less make it rise! For writing this book, I am indebted to Alex Jack, master writer, his wife Gale for copyediting, and to their apprentices at One Peaceful World Press who typed, edited, and corrected this text including Lynda Shoup. I am also grateful to Lily Kushi who made many of the graceful drawings in this book.

Guy Lalumiere
Becket, Massachusetts
Spring 1993

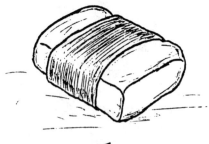

1
Mochi

Mochi is made from sweet brown rice, a variety of rice which is very sweet and sticky. The rice is soaked, pressure-cooked or steamed, then pounded and shaped into cakes. Once dried, these cakes can be sliced and fried, boiled, baked, or steamed. Mixed with seeds, nuts or vegetables, they make delicious dishes. When dried properly, they can keep for months without refrigeration, and can be cooked ready to eat in a few minutes. Mochi makes very handy camping food or snacks.

In Japan, where it originated, mochi is known to increase physical strength and stamina. For these reasons, it is easy to understand why mochi is said to promote longevity. It is used to correct anemia and intestinal weakness and to increase strength and milk supply in lactating mothers.

There is an important symbolism attached to mochi. It is often offered at shrines. It is always the central part of many celebrations. For example, during a celebration for boys and girls, it is given as a symbol of endurance through the future difficulties of life. During the Japanese New Year's celebrations (*O-Sho-gatsu*) from January 1st to January 20th, a special kind of mochi (*Ka gami-mochi*) is used as the central ornament at the entrance of every house, just like the Christmas wreath is used in the West.

Last year, I was invited to celebrate New Year's Day (*O-Sho-gatsu*) with a Japanese family, and greatly enjoyed taking

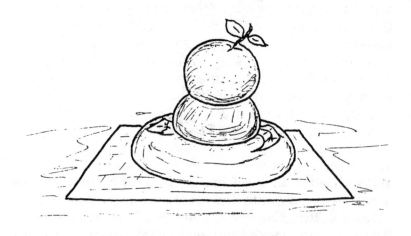

Ka gami-mochi served at New Year's in Japan.

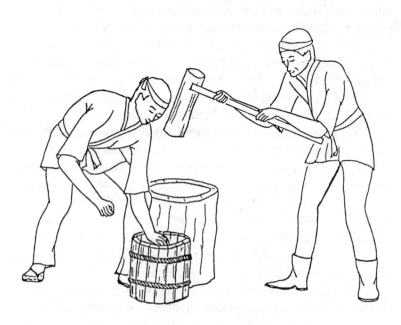

Traditional pounding of mochi in the Far East.

part in their tradition of preparing mochi. On New Year's Day, the grandparents welcome all their children and grandchildren for the celebration. While one woman steams the sweet rice, the men set up a very large mortar (sometimes made of a large hollowed piece of granite or log) and two or three wooden mallets. When the sweet rice is ready, it is transferred to the moistened mortar which holds 15-20 cups. Three men, each holding a moistened mallet, take turns pounding the rice. This requires very careful timing. Occasionally, a woman will check the rice to see if it is sufficiently pounded. With three men at work, it takes about ten minutes to make beautifully soft and silky mochi.

The entire morning is spent making mochi in this way, with the occasional sake-break every once in a while! When the rice is pounded, the grandmother has it brought to a table where she and the other women present shape it into small cakes which are dusted with flour (arrowroot, rice, or other). These mochi are then left to dry, and will be eaten throughout January at different festivities. Some are set aside to be used as New Year's decorations, the equivalent of our Christmas decorations. To make these, a small round mochi, sometimes colored green, is placed on a large white one, and topped with a tangerine. This decoration is placed at the entrance of every Japanese home, where it is left for two weeks and then eaten.

The day after New Year's, a special soup called *o-zoni* is made in the morning. It contains a few pieces of the mochi made the previous day. In southern and western Japan, the soup is clear and light, and the mochi added are round; whereas in the east and north, the soup is thicker and the mochi are square in shape.

Making Mochi

Sweet brown rice contains a high proportion of a type of starch called amylopectic which is responsible for its sticky texture and strong binding quality. This binding power develops when the cooked rice is pounded, kneaded, or ground.

The texture of mochi becomes softer and smoother when it is pounded, and the longer the pounding the better. A mill can also be used to grind the mochi which will become smooth and elastic if it is then kneaded.

Although it is sometimes called glutinous rice, there is no gluten in mochi. The binding is caused by the peculiar type of starch in sweet rice, not by protein bonds.

Procedure

One cup of sweet brown rice (7 ounces solid) makes between 8 and 10 ounces (solid) of mochi. The following recipe will make about 1 1/4 lbs.

1. Wash 2 cups of sweet brown rice and soak overnight in 3 1/2 cups water. Or if you wish you can soak the rice up to 24 hours. It will become a little bit softer. Do not use too much water or you will not be able to shape the mochi later. It will be too soft.

2. Either
a) Pressure cook for 45 minutes using a very low flame over a flame tamer. Be careful, sweet rice burns very easily; or
b) Pressure steam. When sweet rice is pressure steamed, it does not absorb more water during cooking. It cooks with only the water it has absorbed during soaking, which is just the right amount of water to make mochi. Also, when you pressure steam, it cooks much more thoroughly and, of course, it does not burn.

To pressure steam, put a vegetable steamer into a pressure cooker and line it with a piece of cheesecloth. Put about 1 inch of water into the pressure cooker. Discard the soaking water and put the soaked rice only on the cheesecloth. Put the lid on and pressure steam for 60 minutes.

3. Turn off the flame and let the pressure come down.

4. For easy pounding, the utensils must be moistened

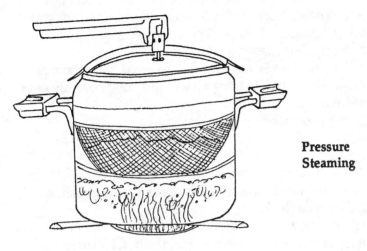

Pressure Steaming

and the rice must be as hot as possible. Remove only as much as you can pound at one time. Keep the remaining rice hot by replacing the lid of the pressure-cooker. Using a *suribachi* and *surikogi*, or a large mortar and pestle, pound the rice for about 15 minutes by holding the mortar between your legs, or have a friend hold the mortar, and re-wetting the pounding implement from time to time. Most of the grains should be crushed and become smooth and sticky.

A Corona Mill can also be used (*see Appendix*). With wet hands, make a ball of sweet rice the size of a baseball. Push it into the mouth of the mill, and grind at a fine setting.

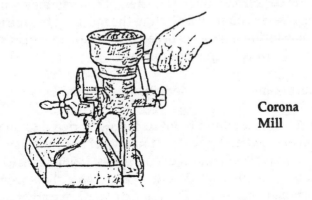

Corona Mill

5. The ground rice must be shaped while it is still hot and moist. When it cools down, it hardens and dries, making it difficult to knead and shape. There are many different ways to shape mochi. For example, you can:

a) Wet your hands and knead a fist sized ball of mochi into a small round loaf. Let dry on a floured plate or a sheet of nori seaweed.

b) Dust your hands with sweet brown rice flour or arrowroot flour and shape into round loaves. Let dry on a floured plate.

c) Sprinkle a baking sheet with water or arrowroot flour and spread the mochi on all the surface of the baking sheet, about 1/2 - 1 inch thick.

d) Dust a large soup bowl with sweet rice flour or arrowroot flour and pour the mochi into the bowl. Flatten and let dry in the refrigerator overnight. The next morning, turn the bowl upside down, and tap the bowl lightly to remove the mochi.

When mochi is shaped into a round loaf, it tends to flatten as it dries. Smaller loaves will keep their shape better than bigger ones. If it flattens, you can reshape it round as long as it does not dry out. To help it keep a nice rounded shape, you can wrap the sides of the loaf with a piece of wax paper.

6) If you don't wish to eat the mochi immediately, and don't mind missing a treat, let the mochi dry overnight in a cool, dry place. The next morning, turn them upside down and let the bottom dry out completely. This way they will keep for weeks. You may also store the mochi in the refrigerator. Avoid storing in plastic, because the trapped moisture promotes the development of molds.

Mochi can also be made with other ingredients. For example:

a) When you pound or grind the sweet rice, add about 1 teaspoon of dried and powdered mugwort per cup of sweet rice. It is available in Japanese food stores. If you want to make your own, pick only the tip of a growing shoot from a mugwort plant and dry it. Do not use older leaves that have a dark green color. They are too bitter. Mugwort colors the mochi green. You can also use *ao-nori* flakes if you cannot find mugwort.

b) Instead of mugwort you can add 1/2 - 1 teaspoon of dried and ground saffron or shiso leaves. They make red mochi.

c) Cook 1 cup of sweet brown rice and one cup millet or brown rice together. Pound as for regular mochi.

d) You can add wet ingredients, but be careful. The mochi will spoil faster. For example, you can add raisins or currants when you pound the sweet rice. But these mochi will not keep very well.

e) If you can find glutinous millet, you can use it instead of sweet rice. It makes excellent mochi.

f) Sesame seeds, almonds, walnuts, or chestnuts can also be added when grinding the sweet rice.

In some areas, sweet rice is not available. Mochi can be made with regular rice. Choose the most sticky variety available. You can also sprout regular brown rice for 3-4 days, pressure cook it for 45 minutes, and pound it into mochi.

Finally, mochi can also be made with sprouted spelt or wheat which has been sprouted for two days, cooked for 1 hour, and pounded. Oats can also be used. It has been made into cakes for travelers in northern European countries for a long time.

Large Quantity

On a large scale, mochi is made by grinding the cooked sweet rice with a commercial electric meat grinder. Since it is very sticky, special equipment or ingenuity is used to package it into plastic bags. It must be refrigerated immediately. It cannot keep more than two weeks in a sealed plastic bag unless it is frozen.

One pound of sweet brown rice (at 13 percent moisture) can make about 1 pound 6 ounces of mochi (at 36 percent moisture).

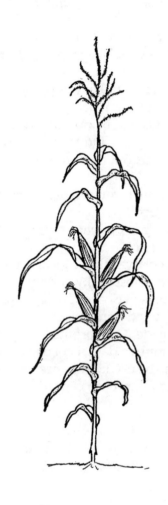

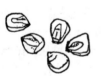

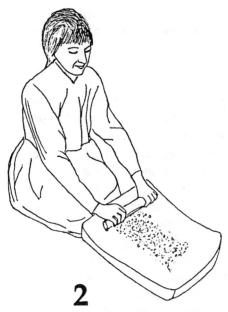

2
Corn Masa

Corn has been the staple of American Indians for many centuries. It is a gift of the Gods, the central pivot of all American Indian civilizations. It is present in all aspects of daily life, from birth to death, and it features in many ceremonies.

The Indians have grown many different varieties of corn over the centuries, and many new varieties have been produced this last century. They are classified in four families. *Dent corn* is the most easily available. Its name comes from the presence of a small dent on top of the grain. It is a starchy grain. *Flint corn* is said to be the true Indian corn. It is smaller than dent corn and cooks faster. It has a very pleasant taste. *Popcorn* is the type well known. It can also be cooked like the other corns. Finally, *sweet corn* is a new variety of corn that is devoid of starch. It cannot be used for the following recipe.

Corn masa is a dough ("masa" in Spanish), which is made of whole corn kernels cooked with wood ash and ground. Called "nixtamal" in ancient Mexican, it is the most versatile way to eat corn. It is the base for hominy, arepas, tacos, tortillas, tamales (corn masa and vegetables wrapped in a corn husk and baked), as well as many other dishes from Native America.

Corn masa is also the most wholesome and nutritious way to eat corn. Although corn contains niacin and amino acids, these nutrients cannot be fully absorbed by humans when the grain is eaten on its own. When cooked with wood ash or limestone, however, a chemical reaction takes place which releases the niacin and modifies the proteins, making them available for human digestion.

Limestone is the underground accumulated debris of algae and crustaceans from ancient oceans. A few centuries ago, Indians used roasted and crushed mussel shells which contain limestone for the same purpose. Corn cooked with wood ash or shells has been a staple of the Indian diet ever since the discovery of this cooking process many centuries ago. In countries where corn was eaten as a staple without the use of wood ash, people developed nutritional deficiencies such as kwashiorkor (vitamin and protein deficiency) in Africa, and pellagra (vitamin B deficiency) in the southern United States.

The niacin in corn is found on the skin of its kernel. During cooking, the wood ashes soften the skin which permits the kernel to cook and soften. The niacin is then released and absorbed into the kernel. After cooking, the skins dissolve and are washed away with the wood ashes.

Procedure

This recipe will make 4 pounds of masa.

1. Wash 4 cups of corn kernels. You can use dent, flint, corn, or popcorn.

2. Put about 1 cup of wood ashes on a piece of thin cotton, fold the corners, and tie to form a small bag. This way the wood ashes will be easier to wash away when the corn is

cooked. Oak ashes are best. Make sure the ashes are clean (no paint, nails, etc.) and have been sifted.

The quantity of ashes needed depends on the type of corn used and the strength of the wood ashes (quantity of alkali in the ashes). One cup of wood ashes will soften the skins of 3 to 5 cups of corn kernels. Experiment with the corn and ashes that are available to you until you find the minimum quantity of wood ashes needed to dissolve all the skins of the corn.

3. Bring 8 cups of water to a boil in a pressure cooker.

4. Add the 4 cups of corn and the small bag of wood ashes. Bring to a boil again.

5. Turn off the flame, cover, and let soak overnight. It takes between 2 and 8 hours to soften the skins. Overnight is the maximum needed.

6. After soaking, inspect the kernels. Some varieties of corn have a very thin skin that dissolve easily. If the skins are dissolved, cook only for a short time (next step).

7. If the skins are not dissolved, turn on the flame and bring up to pressure. Lower the flame and cook for 45-75 minutes. Some varieties of corn cook quickly, others take longer. Cook only until the kernels become crunchy but not mushy. The skins should become gelatinous and detach easily from the kernels. Dent corn takes about 60 minutes of cooking, popcorn about 70 to 75 minutes, and flint corn between 15 and 30 minutes.

8. After soaking and cooking, inspect the kernels. The skins should be floating in the cooking water as thin gelatinous membranes. The kernels should be soft but still whole. If the kernels are broken open with the skin still attached, you need to use more wood ashes and soak longer.

But be careful; do not overcook. The purpose of this cooking is to dissolve the skins only, not cook the corn. If you cook too long, the ashes will penetrate into the kernels and they will turn gray. You will not be able to wash them off. Good masa should be bright yellow and should not taste of ashes. Some varieties of corn require very little cooking. You must experiment and find out.

Discard the small bag of ashes and transfer the corn in a colander into your sink. Wash the corn under running water and rub the corn between your hands to remove all the skins and any wood ash. Rinse until the corn becomes bright yellow and the slippery texture of the wood ashes disappears.

9. There are two different ways to do the next step: one is quicker, the other one is longer but makes a nicer masa.

a) *Quick way:* put the washed corn into a pressure cooker, add water about 4 fingers above the level of corn, add 4 pinches of salt, and pressure cook on a low flame for 15 to 30 minutes. Again, do not overcook. If they are left to cook too long, the kernels will become too soft. The masa will be too wet. The grains must become soft and mushy.

b) *Long way:* put the washed corn into a pot, add water about 4 fingers above the level of corn, and let soak for 8 hours.

10. Strain the cooking water into a bowl and set aside. Grind the kernels in a Corona Mill at a fine setting. The Corona Mill, made in South America where corn is eaten as staple food, is available at most natural food and hardware stores. A mortar and pestle can also be used to grind the corn until a soft dough is obtained. Collect the dough into a baking pan.

11. Use the cooking water set aside earlier to wet your hands and knead the dough. Add a little bit of water as you knead to adjust the consistency. The dough must not be too mushy or sticky. It should become elastic. When sufficiently kneaded, cover with a damp towel and refrigerate. Or flatten on the baking pan to make a smooth surface and let dry overnight. The masa will set and can be cut into squares with a knife. It can also be shaped into balls to make tacos, tortillas, and arepas. Vegetables and seasonings can be kneaded in.

You can incorporate a little more water if a smoother consistency is desired. When sufficiently dried, corn masa keeps for 1-2 weeks in the refrigerator, but will spoil easily if wrapped in plastic.

Hominy

Whole cooked corn kernels (step 8) can be eaten as they are without grinding. They are called hominy and make delicious dishes. Cook them in soup or with other grains or vegetables until they become completely soft.

They can also be stored for future use. Put the corn with some cooking water into mason jars and pressure steam about 30 minutes.

Cooking Corn with Lime

If wood ash is not available, corn can be cooked with lime. Between one and two ounces of food grade lime is needed per pound of corn (about 2 cups). But lime is a very strong alkaline. If you use lime, do not boil (step #7). Also, the corn must be washed thoroughly (step #8) to remove all traces of lime. Lime is not edible.

Tortillas

Take a ping pong ball sized portion of masa and flatten using a floured tortilla press or put between two layers of wax paper and roll flat with a rolling pin. Heat and lightly oil a skillet. Cook one side. Then turn over and cook the other side until some brown spots appear and the edges of the tortilla curl up.

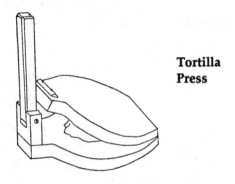

**Tortilla
Press**

Arepas

Chop onions, carrots, parsley, or other vegetables finely and incorporate into a small ball of masa. Shape into a croquette and pan-fry. These can be served with a shoyu-ginger sauce, a creamy sauce, or an endless variety of ways.

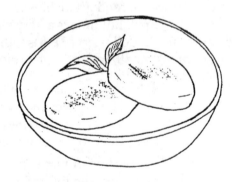

Arepas

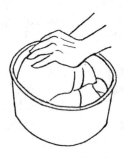

3
Seitan and Fu

Both seitan and fu are made from gluten, the protein of wheat. They were first made many centuries ago in China and Japan by vegetarian Buddhist monks as a substitute for meat. George Ohsawa coined the word "seitan" (though the food was very traditional), and "fu" is also Japanese in origin. Seitan is also known as wheat gluten or wheat meat. It was made traditionally in Europe, as well as by the Seventh Day Adventists in America who are vegetarians.

Seitan and fu are made from a bread dough which is washed in water to remove the starch and bran. What remains is a very elastic mass of threads which does not dissolve in water. It is the gluten, the protein of wheat. When making bread dough, it is the gluten which gives plasticity and elasticity to the dough. The gluten is also responsible for its spongy texture: bread is made of particles of starch embedded in a network of gluten fibers.

Both seitan and fu are very nutritious, and a good source of protein. One cup of gluten contains 70-75 grams of protein. Cooked seitan looks very much like beef, while fu somewhat resembles crackers. They are delicious cooked with vegetables as stew, deep-fried, or in baked dishes. Fu also goes very well in soups. Seitan is heavier, stronger, and is well suited for cold winter days. Fu is very light and easy to digest, even by children. It is more suited for hot summer days.

They are very easy to make at home. Seitan will keep at least one week in the refrigerator, while fu keeps indefinitely when dried.

When making seitan and fu, the most important point is choosing the proper kind of flour. There are basically two varieties of wheat: hard and soft. Hard wheat contains more protein than soft wheat, and is also harder, and usually has a dark red color. It is used for making bread. Soft wheat is usually cream-colored and contains less protein and more starch. It is used for pastry-making.

Hard wheat should be used to make seitan and fu. There are two types of hard wheat: hard spring wheat is planted in the spring and harvested in the summer, while hard winter wheat is planted in the fall and harvested the following spring. Hard spring wheat contains a little more protein than hard winter wheat, which is higher in minerals.

Type of wheat	Protein (gm/100)	Uses
Hard spring wheat	16.5	bread
Hard winter wheat	15.3	seitan and fu
Soft winter wheat	11.2	
Soft spring wheat	12.4	pastries

Seitan

Seitan is very easy to make at home in a short time. It is also inexpensive and keeps for at least one week in the refrigerator.

The following recipe will make about 6 cups of seitan, which is approximately a one week's supply for a family. As a general rule, you should be able to make a ball of gluten of half of the size of the dough you made with the flour. And it should give you a ball of seitan of the same size as the dough you started with. When you wash the dough, about half of it remains as gluten. And when you cook gluten, it nearly doubles in size.

1. Put 8 cups of flour into a large bowl.
• You can use whole wheat bread flour, unbleached white flour, or a combination of both. If you use only whole wheat bread flour, the seitan will be a little firmer, whereas with unbleached white flour, it will be more light and elastic. You will also obtain a little more seitan when using white flour. To obtain intermediate texture, use a combination of both and mix them thoroughly.
• Do not use all purpose flour. It is made of half hard wheat and half soft wheat.
• If the flour you use has a low content of gluten, you may add some gluten flour to it to increase its strength (available in natural food stores). But use as little as possible. Seitan made from gluten flour has a rubbery texture and an inferior taste.

2. Add 4 cups cold water and mix thoroughly. Then let rest 2-3 minutes.
• The gluten network begins to form when the flour absorbs water. And that takes between 5 and 15 minutes. At the beginning, kneading is of very little use.
Fill a small bowl with cold water, dip your hands into the water, and knead the dough for 4-5 minutes. From time to time, dip your hands into the water to keep them wet and prevent the dough from sticking. Then, let rest 2-3 minutes.
• Kneading with wet hands is much easier. The dough never becomes hard and dry, and it does not stick.
Knead again for 4-5 minutes, always keeping your hands wet. The dough will become very smooth, elastic, and slippery as you knead. Then let it rest for 2-3 minutes.

• As the flour progressively absorbs water, the two main proteins of wheat, gliadin (which has a positive electric charge) and glutanin (which has a negative electric charge) combine together to form tangled threads of gluten

• Kneading stretches these threads and aligns them with each other. It also stimulates the formation of a long, elastic continuous network of gluten fibers.

• Alternating periods of kneading and resting make a gluten which is very smooth and elastic. (It is also much easier to make a dough this way). When a dough is kneaded continuously for 10-15 minutes, the gluten becomes very stiff, and difficult to knead. The actual number of strokes used to knead has very little to do with the development of the gluten.

Knead one last time for 2-3 minutes. The dough will become nicely round, firm and elastic. Cover the dough with cold water and let it rest for one hour.

• The gluten network develops when the dough is resting, not when it is kneaded. Take note of the changes in the texture of the dough after each period of rest. The complete process of formation of gluten takes about one hour.

• This method of kneading can also be used to make bread doughs which will rise very easily (but don't cover with water).

3. Put the bowl containing the dough into the sink and knead it gently in its soaking water until it turns milky white. This is the starch dissolving in the water. Put this starchy water into a large pot (about 3-4 gallons). Fill the bowl with enough hot water to cover the dough and gently knead again. More starch and some bran will dissolve. Transfer the water again to the large pot. Repeat these steps four or five times, alternating with cold and hot water. The dough will progressively become more elastic, and threads of gluten will appear. Wash the dough until it becomes a mass of elastic threads firmly bound together. If, during this process, the dough begins falling apart, the wheat used did not have strong gluten. In this case, do not use hot water. Wash out the starch as gently as possible, and put the dough in the refrigerator over-

night, covered with water. It will have become firmer the next day and you can continue washing it to make seitan.

4. Next, hold the mass of gluten in your hands under running water, and stretch it to wash away more starch. Leave some starch in the gluten, but not too much. If too much starch is removed, the seitan will lack flavor; yet, if too much remains, the seitan will be doughy, like dumplings.
You should have about 3 cups of gluten.

5. In a large pot, bring 16-20 cups of water to a boil. Break the mass of gluten into ball-sized pieces half the size of your fist, shape it into round balls and boil for about 15 minutes, until the balls rise to the surface and float. You can also shape the gluten into a cylinder by rolling it in a cotton towel, then boiling it for 15 minutes. The gluten can be molded into any shape desired. If boiled vigorously, the gluten will double in volume and become very light, whereas if simply simmered, it will expand less and be firmer. After boiling, remove the balls of cooked gluten from the water and allow to cool. Turn off the flame.

6. To the same water, add the following seasonings:
• one 6-inch piece of kombu seaweed
• 2 or 3 shiitake mushrooms
• 1/2 teaspoon grated ginger or
  2 bay leaves or
  any other desired seasoning
• shoyu soy sauce
  for mild seitan: 1/2 -3/4 cup
  for strong seitan: 1 - 1 1/2 cups
There should be about twice as much liquid as gluten. Let the kombu and shiitake rehydrate 30 minutes and simmer 15 minutes before adding the shoyu soy sauce.
Bring to a boil and drop the cooked gluten into the broth. Simmer for about one hour if the broth is mildly salted. If using a stronger broth, simmer for 3-4 hours, preferably using a heavy cast-iron pot and adding water when needed. The longer seitan is cooked, the firmer it becomes.

7. Transfer the seitan and broth into a bowl, allow it to cool, and then refrigerate. It will keep at least a week. You should obtain about 6-8 cups of seitan.

8. As an alternative, you can cook the balls of gluten directly into the broth and skip step #5 if you do not wish to shape the gluten in a special way. Simply make balls about the size of your fist and cook for 1 1/2 hours.

You can also steam the gluten on a vegetable steamer over 1 inch of water in a pot. It will cook very softly this way.

Raw gluten can be stored in the refrigerator covered with water for a few days. It can be used as dumplings in soups. Wrapped around carrots or burdock and stewed or deep-fried, it makes delicious dishes. After a few hours of rest in water, it becomes very soft and elastic. It can be stretched on an oiled baking pan, filled with vegetables, and covered with another sheet of gluten. It is baked slowly and makes a very filling winter dish.

9. The washing water containing the starch and the bran, which was set aside earlier in a large pot, can also be further used. The starch should be allowed to settle overnight in a cool place. Then discard the water, remove the starch, and allow it to dry in the sun or in an oven at low temperature. This dried starch can be used as a thickener in the same way as kuzu and arrowroot, or added to breads and pastries. The starch water can also be made into syrup or an amazake-like drink.

Fu

The procedure for making fu is much the same as that for seitan except that the end-product is dried and resembles crackers. Fu can be used in the same recipes as seitan.

The fu sold in natural food stores is made in Japan where special equipment and techniques are used. For example, in making *kuruma fu* or *zenryu fu*, the round type, the dough is washed and wrapped around a rod and toasted in the oven. Three more layers of dough are added and toasted successively. The cylinder formed is then steamed, cut, and dried. These types of fu are difficult to produce at home, but an easier recipe follows. Once dried, it keeps for many months and can be used just as the store-bought fu.

1. Make a dough as described for seitan.

2. Wash the dough as with seitan, but continue with one of the following variations:
    a) For fu with a whole-wheat texture, do not wash away all the starch and bran.
    b) For a light-textured fu, wash away all the starch and bran. Squeeze the water out of the gluten, put it in a bowl, and knead in unbleached white flour (2 cups of flour per 4 cups of gluten). It will take some time and kneading to incorporate all the flour. You should obtain a flexible white dough. Instead of white flour, sweet brown rice flour can also be used.

3. Allow the dough to sit for half an hour in a bowl filled with warm water.
    N.B. There are two key factors in making good fu:
    a) First, the gluten must be completely relaxed. When gluten is worked, it becomes tense and elastic. To make light fu, the gluten must be quite soft and must not shrink when stretched. When cooked, it must expand as much as possible.
    b) Second, the dough must be very soft and wet to facilitate the expansion of gluten when it is cooked.

4. Using a pump bottle (the type used to water plants or wash windows), spray water on a cookie sheet. Form dough into 1-inch lumps and place on the sheet, leaving enough space between them to allow for expansion. Then sprinkle once again with water. The lumps can be made in various shapes and sizes (e.g., marbles or breadsticks). However, avoid making them too large as they won't cook properly.

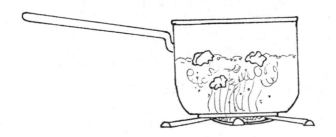

5. Bake at 500 degrees F. on the lower shelf for 3-4 minutes, until puffed up. Then transfer to the upper shelf for a further 3-4 minutes until golden brown.

6. Remove from the oven and transfer the fu to a metal tray. They won't stick to the sheets if sufficient water has been used.

7. Turn off the heat, and return the trays of fu to the oven. Allow them to dry out completely (overnight). This way, they will keep for months.

8. Fu can also be boiled. Simply drop small lumps of the dough into boiling water. Boil until the lumps rise to the surface and float (5-10 minutes). Thin sheets of dough can also be boiled this way. When cooked, remove from the boiling water and dry on a towel. Keep refrigerated.

9. Small balls of boiled fu are also delicious pickled in miso. After boiling, dry the fu with a towel, and place in a container filled with miso. Leave for 3-6 days. If they are left longer, the pieces of fu will become hard.

10. The small lumps of dough are very tasty deep-fried as tempura.

11. Uncooked dough can be kept up to seven days if covered with water and refrigerated.

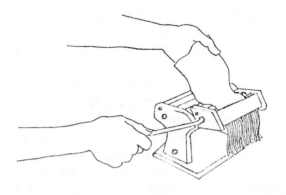

4
Noodles

I love noodles. I can live on them. They are one of the foods I have the most pleasure making and experimenting with. The basic recipe for noodles is very simple. With a little bit of practice, they can be made in no time and eaten fresh. Even on the first try, homemade noodles have a taste and texture that surpass the best store-bought varieties. If you can grind your own flour to make your own dough, they will be even better. There is only one thing you must be careful with: you must make a dough that has just the right consistency. It is much easier to work with, and it makes much better noodles. You will develop a feel for it easily after maybe two or three trials.

There is a wide variety of noodles made today. They can be divided in two categories: the Western type which origi-nated in southern Europe and spread all over the world and the Eastern type which originated in China and Japan. The differences in these two types of noodles reflect the particu-larities of these two cultures.

The Western noodles, as developed in Italy, are made of

durum wheat which contains a high proportion of gluten. It is gound into a flour called semolina, refined (bran and germ removed), and enriched. In natural foods stores, unrefined whole-wheat noodles are available. A dough is made from that flour and either eggs (four large eggs per pound of flour) or salt (1 percent) and water are added. This dough is fed into an extruder which is a mill that mixes the dough and forces it through holes in front of which small knives rotate. The size and shape of these holes determines the forms of the noodles.

The Eastern noodles, as made in Japan today, can be divided in two types: *udon* and *somen* which are made of various proportions of different soft wheat flours and *soba*, which are made of different proportions of buckwheat and wheat flour. To make these noodles, the flour is mixed with water and salt, kneaded, and the resulting dough is left to rest for a few hours. Next, it is rolled into a thin, long sheet, folded, and then cut into noodles with a heavy knife. This process is more gentle than the extrusion method. The use of softer varieties of wheat and the absence of eggs give noodles a very delicate texture. In Western countries, noodles are chewy, and they are usually eaten with herbs, tomato sauce, and oil. In Japan, they make noodles very soft and some of them are very thin. They are eaten often with a salty broth.

When I first tried the Japanese noodles, I was very pleased with their fine texture. They are made of different combinations of whole wheat and white flour. And they are cut in different ways. Some are cut more wide; they are used in warming, hearty dishes. Some others are cut more thin; they make very refreshing summer meals. They are sometimes served in a bed of ice cubes with a salty and sour dip, during the hot, humid days of summer in Japan. In that country, they have small udon and soba restaurants on every street corner and in every train station. The noodles are usually served in a piping hot broth seasoned with soy sauce, shiitake, bonito (fish) flakes, and mirin (sweet rice wine), and garnished with tofu, wakame sea vegetable, vegetables, or tempura (deep-fried vegetables). When you order them, the cooks prepare your order in one minute in front of you. Some restaurants specialize in udon and soba. The cook makes the dough, rolls, and cuts it into noodles by hand, and cooks them in front of customers very quickly. When I first saw these noodle makers, I was amazed by their dexterity and the speed. So I tried making my own, and I found out that it could be done simply, maybe not as good as the noodles made by a professional, but still very reasonable, and much cheaper than the store-bought varieties.

A Noodle Glossary

To help untangle the Japanese noodle lingo, following is a brief description of the names and composition of the most common noodles made. (There are actually hundreds of variations.)

Udon Thick, flat (1/8 to 1/4 inch) wheat noodles, available in white, whole wheat, or a combination of both.

Tsuru Udon Wide, 60 percent whole wheat and 40 percent white.

Whole Wheat Udon Wide 100 percent whole wheat.

Brown Rice Udon 75 percent wheat flour (white and whole wheat) and 25 percent brown rice flour.

Somen Thin wheat noodles, available in white, whole wheat, or a combination of both. They cook more quickly than udon.

Tsuru Somen 100 percent white flour.

Hiya Mugi or Whole Wheat Somen 100 percent whole-wheat flour made from soft wheat.

Soba Thin, square section, buckwheat and wheat flour noodles.

Ito Soba Very thin, 40 percent buckwheat, 60 percent wheat flours.

Various Soba Thin, square, made of 70 to 100 percent buckwheat flour, with 0 to 30 percent wheat flour.

Jinenjo Soba Buckwheat and wheat flour and grated Japanese mountain potato.

Cha Soba Buckwheat and wheat flour and green tea; eaten cold.

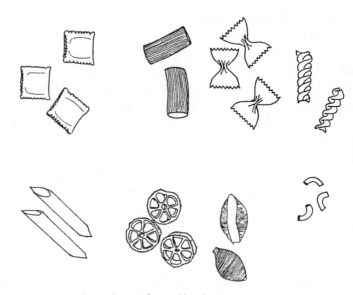

A variety of noodle shapes.

Yomogi Soba Buckwheat and wheat flours and mugwort (a green herb).

Ramen Square, packaged, curly type of noodles. Of Chinese origin, very popular today in Japan. Available in natural foods stores in whole wheat and many different flavors (for example, mushroom, garlic, etc.).

Kuzu Noodles Made with kuzu (a powdered white root) and water (about 8 tablespoons of kuzu per 2 cups of water), heated to thicken, poured into a pan, and chilled. The kuzu jelly is then cut in thin noodles.

There are many cookbooks available which describe the procedure for making egg noodles. But very few explain how to make the Far Eastern varieties. Following is a descrption of the method I use to make udon and soba. I experimented with many combinations of flours and methods. Some are easier to make, some are more challenging. Rolling and cutting requires a bit of practice. But if you want, you can use one of the small hand-cranked machines that roll and cut noodles easily. They are available at cooking supply stores.

Making the Dough

Making noodles at home is not too difficult. And once you have acquired the feel of it, they can be made very quickly. The taste and texture of freshly made noodles can be adjusted by changing the proportions of ingredients.

There is almost a limitless combination of ingredients that can be used to make noodles. Many different kinds of flours can be used in different proportions. Some of these are easier to make into noodles; others, such as buckwheat, require more practice. Following is a list of combinations you can try. They are listed in order of difficulty, the easiest at the beginning. They add up to 2 cups of flour which you add to 1/2 cup of water in which 1 teaspoon of salt has been dissolved.

The salt gives strength to the gluten. For 2 cups of flour, you need between 1/2 and 1 level teaspoon of salt. If the wheat flour you use has more gluten, you can use less salt. The first time you make noodles, use 1 level teaspoon of salt to make sure they will not break. The next time, try using less. As you learn to knead your dough more thoroughly and develop a feel for the right consistency, you will be able to reduce the amount of salt and still make strong noodles.

Two cups of flour and 1/2 cup of water will make enough noodles for two meals (10 to 14 ounces of dried noodles) or four soup portions.

If you make a dough that contains buckwheat, use about 3/4 cup of water and heat it before adding it to the flour. It will facilitate the binding of the dough. If you use wet ingredients (like vegetables or jinenjo for jinenjo soba), you must reduce the amount of water you use.

The flour must be ground very fine if you grind your own. Sifting is also recommended. A variety of wheat with a lower content of gluten makes much finer and softer noodles. The dough is easier to knead and roll. For these reasons, a combination of bread wheat and pastry wheat gives better results if the bread wheat flour you use (or the unbleached white flour) has a high content of gluten. Spelt is the very best variety of wheat that can be used to make noodles. Its gluten is very soft and elastic. It makes noodles with a wonderful taste. You don't need to use durum wheat to make noodles. Its gluten is very hard, and it makes very firm noodles. It is used mainly to make noodles which are shaped with an extruder. A dough made from durum wheat is difficult to roll thin; it springs back easily and tears frequently.

If you use buckwheat flour, you must make sure that no large pieces of husks remain. Since buckwheat noodles must be cut very fine, large pieces of husks will weaken the dough and the noodles will break easily. (If you have difficulty with buckwheat, try grinding buckwheat grains which you can buy in natural foods stores; it does not contain husks.)

The same thing may happen with whole wheat noodles if big pieces of bran remain in the flour.

Use either one of these:
* 2 cups unbleached white flour for easy-to-make white noodles; good for light somen noodles
* 1 cup unbleached white flour plus 1 cup whole wheat flour for regular udon
* 1 1/2 cups whole wheat flour plus 1/2 cup unbleached white flour for tsuru udon
* 1 to 1 1/2 cups unbleached white flour plus 1/2 to 1 cup brown rice flour for brown rice udon
* 1 to 1 1/2 cups whole wheat flour plus 1/2 to 1 cup brown rice flour; a bit more difficult to make
* 2 cups spelt flour (whole); the very best whole-wheat noodles there are and easy to make
* 1 cup whole wheat bread flour plus 1 cup whole wheat pastry flour; very good whole wheat noodles
* 1 cup unbleached white flour plus 1 cup buckwheat flour; the easiest buckwheat noodles to make; if cut very fine, they make ito soba
* 1/2 cup unbleached white flour plus 1 1/2 cups buckwheat flour; more difficult. Heat the water and use 3/4 cup.
In Japan, the buckwheat noodles are classified by ratios of buckwheat flour to wheat flour, being written 70/30, 80/20, 90/10, etc. But these measures can only be approximated with

the American system of measures.
- 2 cups buckwheat flour; for a challenging adventure!

Sift and mix the flours thoroughly. You can add many ingredients to the flours to color and flavor the noodles. Different flours can be used with the wheat flour such as corn, oats, soybean, or chickpea flour. Use up to 1/2 cup of any of these for 1 1/2 cups of wheat flour.

About 2 to 3 tablespoons of the following can be puréed or minced and mixed with the water. If the ingredients are wet, reduce the amount of water slightly.
- You can use herbs such as basil, oregano, sage, coriander, thyme, green or red shiso, garlic, or parsley.
- Vegetables such as carrot, squash, or any greens can also be used.
- The cha-soba are made by adding green tea powder to the water. Yomogi soba is made by adding dried mugwort. You can also try green nori flakes.

When you use these ingredients, make sure they are minced or puréed very fine. If the pieces are too big, they will weaken the noodles and they will break easily.

Soba noodles which contain a high proportion of buckwheat flour are more difficult to make since buckwheat has no gluten. To help bind the dough, a variety of Japanese mountain potato (jinenjo or yama imo) can be used to make a variety of noodles called jinenjo soba. For 2 cups of buckwheat flour, grate about 1/2 cup of jinenjo and 1 teaspoon salt and mix into the flour. (You may need to add a little water.) Jinenjo is very mucilaginous and it will help bind the dough. It is available in some natural foods stores and at Japanese specialty stores.

Put all the ingredients into a sturdy wooden bowl and slowly add the water while mixing with your fingers. Squeeze the mixture firmly between your fingers to incorporate flour and water completely. This is especially important if you make buckwheat noodles. Since buckwheat has no gluten, it requires more mixing to bind properly. Then begin to form into a ball and knead. The proportions of flour and water listed above will make a dough that is a bit too soft to make good noodles. As you knead, you will need to add a little bit of flour. A good noodle dough must have just the right consistency and texture. If it is too dry, it is hard to roll, and the noodles are difficult to dry properly. If it is too soft and sticky, it is hard to cut, and the noodles break when you hang them to dry. They may also break when you cook them. It is when you knead the dough that you adjust the consistency by adding more or less flour. Since different flours absorb water differently, it is not possible to give exact proportions. Knead the dough as you would knead a bread dough, but put your bowl on a low table so you can use all the strength of your arms. A noodle dough is more stiff than a bread dough. At the beginning, it will break apart, but progressively it will bind and form a cohesive dough. After a few minutes of kneading, it should form a ball a little bit tacky. Add just a little bit of flour and keep kneading. It will form a nice smooth and shiny ball after ten minutes of kneading. It must not stick any more, but on the other hand, it must not crack when you knead it. If it does, you added too much flour. You can try a Japanese method: wrap your dough into a plastic bag, put it on the floor, and knead it for 5 to 10 minutes with your heels! That is the ultimate method to make the finest udon.

To make very thin somen that do not break, the dough must be kneaded vigorously to develop a strong gluten, and help the flour absorb the water completely. It also makes noodles with a very soft and silky texture.

The consistency of your dough determines how easy it will be to roll, cut, dry, and cook your noodles. If your dough is too dry, it will be difficult to roll, and the noodles may break when you dry or cook them. If it is too soft, it will be difficult to cut; the noodles will stick together. They will break when you hang them to dry, and they may break when you cook them. As you practice making noodles, you will be able to judge easily how much flour to add to obtain the right consistency. Until then, you can use one of the small noodle makers that roll and cut noodles easily. With practice, though, you will probably find out that you can roll and cut noodles more quickly by hand.

After kneading, the dough must rest at least one hour to

complete the formation of the gluten. Cover your dough with a damp towel and let it rest between 1 and 3 hours. After 1 hour, you may knead again a few minutes and let rest at least 30 minutes. It is ready to roll when it has become a bit "springy," sticky, and has the consistency of firm putty.

As an alternative, you can wrap your dough into a moist cotton towel and into a plastic bag and put in the refrigerator overnight. It will become very smooth, elastic, and will be very easy to roll the next day. You can also make a large batch of dough that you keep in the refrigerator and use only a portion at a time.

Rolling

Next, dust your counter or a wooden board and a rolling pin, and knead your dough a few more times. If you had your dough in the refrigerator, take it out, and let it warm up a few hours before using . You can, if you wish, wrap the dough again into a plastic bag and knead it with your feet for 5 to 10 minutes.

Then cut the dough in two portions and leave one aside, covered with a damp towel. Flatten the other portion on your dusted countertop. With the rolling pin, roll it from the center toward the periphery to make an oval about the size of your

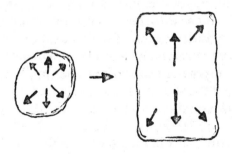

hand. Turn it over and around 90 degrees and roll following the diagram.

Roll a few times in the directions indicated, turn over, rotate 90 degrees, and roll again following the same directions. As you proceed, the oval will stretch into a rectangle of approximately 8 by 16 inches. Apply an even pressure on the rolling pin as you flatten the dough. You must make a thin sheet with a uniform thickness.With your hands, rub the sheet to feel for parts that are too thick or too thin, and correct by rolling more or less.

From time to time, add a little bit of flour on the surface of the dough and rub it gently. It should not stick to the counter or the rolling pin. If it does, you did not use enough flour when you made your dough. But if the edge of the dough tears and cracks, it is too dry. It will be difficult to roll thin. Experts say that you should roll a noodle dough thin enough to be able to read a newspaper through it. I have not succeeded yet, but am working on it!

Resting

When you are finished rolling the first portion into a long thin sheet, sprinkle a bit of flour on it, rub to make a dry, leathery surface, and turn over. Set aside and roll the second portion in the same way. When you are done, again sprinkle a bit of flour on the sheet, rub, and turn over. From a dough made of two cups of flour, you will make two thin sheets of about 8 by 16 inches. Let them rest for about 10 to 15 minutes to relax the gluten and dry the surfaces. Turn the sheets over a few times, sprinkle some flour, if needed, and rub to make a smooth skin. Check for parts that appear too thin and too thick and correct them. If the sheets tend to tear, either you used too much flour, or you did not knead enough. Buckwheat noodles are more brittle; they must be kneaded very well, since buckwheat does not contain gluten. It is the starch that ensures the binding of buckwheat noodles (plus the proportions of wheat flour you used).

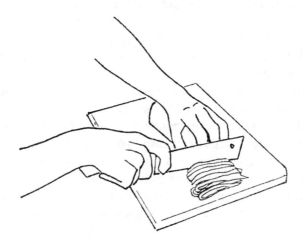

Cutting

To cut noodles more easily, try to get a big, heavy knife with a straight cutting edge. A Chinese chopping knife works well. If you do not have one, you can still use a smaller knife, but make sure the cutting edge is as straight as possible.

Dust the two sheets of dough generously to prevent them from sticking together and put them one over the other in front of you with the narrow side going away from you.

Starting at one end, cut narrow strips (1/8 inch to 1/4 inch) straight down. Do not seesaw or turn your knife. Push the cut noodles aside, separate them, and keep cutting more. It takes a bit of practice to cut very thin noodles. At the beginning, try cutting noodles about the width of your little finger. Lightly toss the cut noodles to prevent them from sticking together. You may sprinkle a bit of flour on them if you wish. Do not compare your noodles with the store-bought varieties. They are all made with precision machinery. Be fair!

Noodles Made with a Machine

When you first make noodles, you may find it a bit difficult to roll the dough thin enough, and cut the noodles very fine. In cookware stores, you can find manual pasta machines that roll and cut the noodles with a few turns of a small hand crank. The machine is made of two parts. The first is a pair of steel rollers that can roll strips of dough of about 6 by 18 inches. The distance between the rollers in adjustable. You simply pass your strips of dough between the rollers a few times and make it thinner every time by changing the adjustment. The second part is a set of detachable noodle cutters. They come in many different sizes of cutting, from the thin somen, to spaghetti, udon, lasagna, and ravioli. You still need to let the sheets of dough rest 15 minutes before cutting.

It takes a bit longer to make noodles with this small machine than by hand, but the noodles always look good.

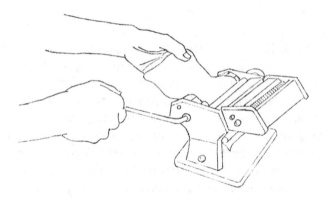

Drying

If you do not want to cook them right away, you can dry the noodles by hanging them on a clothes hanger or a noodle rack (available at cookware stores). To dry properly, noodles should be left to dry in a place that has just the right humidity. They are usually made in areas (Italy or Japan) that are humid. They take 2 to 3 days to dry in these climates. If the air is dry, the noodles will dry more quickly, but they will bend as they dry. Noodles bend if the outside does not dry uniformly, and if it dries much more quickly than the inside. For homemade noodles, this should not be a problem. You can, if you wish, set them in a circle on your dusted counter and let them dry as they are.

If the air is too humid, they may ferment. Gas pockets produced by the fermentation will form in the noodles and they will break into pieces.

In noodle factories, after being cut with machines, the noodles are stored in a room at controlled humidity and temperature. At the beginning of the drying period, they are ventilated with dry air for a short time to dry the surface of the noodles uniformly and prevent bending. Then they are left to dry 15 to 20 hours more.

Cooking

To cook properly, noodles must be boiled in a large amount of water. Put about 4 quarts of water into a pot and bring to a boil. Then grab the freshly cut noodles and put them, a few at a time, into the boiling water so it does not stop boiling. With a chopstick, stir gently to keep the noodles from sticking together. Lower the flame to medium, and let boil for a few minutes. Stir from time to time with chopsticks. Depending how thick you have made your noodles, they will cook in 2 to 5 minutes. Be careful not to overcook. Watch buckwheat noodles carefully. They are difficult to cook and they break easily. They also cook very quickly.

Taste one from time to time to test for doneness. When cooked enough, transfer the noodles into a colander and rinse with cold water to stop cooking and prevent the noodles from sticking together. Toss them around and drain any excess water. They are ready to eat in a broth or with other dishes.

If you cook soba noodles, the cooking liquid makes an excellent broth by itself, seasoned with soy sauce, ginger, nori flakes, or scallions. It is called *soba-yu* in Japan. In soba restaurants, it is always served with the dish of soba, during the meal or at the end.

The cooking water from udon can be used to make soups or cook vegetables. It contains some of the nutrients and the salt of the noodles.

If your noodles don't look like noodles at all, but more like an indescribable culinary oddity, here are some of the reasons:

• Curly noodles: too strong gluten or dough that is too stiff

• Broken noodles: too weak gluten or not enough salt or fermentation (too slow drying); also pieces of bran or ingredients that are too coarse

• Brittle noodles: not enough gluten or they dried too quickly

• Chewy noodles: rolled too thick or not cooked enough

• Noodles that look like wheat cream: beyond hope; add a bit of soy sauce and enjoy anyway

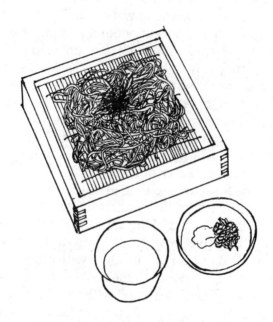

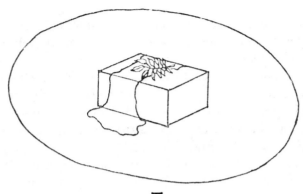

5
Tofu and Soymilk

Introduction

When I started macrobiotics, one of the foods I enjoyed the most was tofu. Silky white soft bean curd has a wonderfully delicate and subtle taste. It is incredibly versatile. I remember when I stayed in Japan, eating in a tofu restaurant where they served full course meals that are composed of twenty or so dishes that all contain tofu, from appetizer to desert. Tofu is also an excellent source of proteins, and very easy to digest. It is eaten daily in many Oriental countries as the main source of protein.

Back then, I had difficulties finding tofu in natural food stores, so I decided to make my own. I found a recipe, gathered the utensils, and tried to make one batch. It was a complete disaster. After hours of painstaking labor, I ended up with just enough tofu to taste two or three morsels of this most delicious, well intentioned, but misguided culinary experience.

But I did not give up! After searching and experimenting, I realized I had made every possible mistake. So I improved my recipe and tried again. Every time I made it, I obtained more and much nicer tofu. For the last three years, the Kushi Institute in Becket has been making tofu according to this method. Every week people comment that this is the best tofu they ever had. There is one simple reason for that: the tofu is freshly made.

Fresh tofu has a wonderful taste and texture. After a few days it becomes hard and bitter or may also turn slightly sour, making it difficult to cook with. Tofu that is more than a week old should never be eaten. Unfortunately, this is the kind of tofu you often find in stores.

At home or in your community, you can make tofu with a unique mellow sweetness which is seldom found in store-bought tofu.

Homemade Tofu

At home, a week's supply of tofu can be made easily in about one hour. The procedure described below is simple. After you have made tofu a few times, you will be able to make it more quickly by planning ahead the different steps of the procedure. You will also be able to cook a simple meal and make your tofu at the same time. Gather the pots and utensils you need, and keep them together always. This way you can set up quickly.

This recipe will make between 3 and 4 pounds of tofu (about one week's supply). Every step of the process has a big influence on the quality and the quantity of tofu you will make. The most common problem encountered when people make tofu for the first time is the small quantity of tofu they end up with after hours of work.

The following procedure explains why this may happen, and how to obtain the highest quantity of tofu possible. It also describes different ways to change the texture and the firmness of the tofu to suit your taste.

You will need:

- 3 cups yellow soybeans
- 5–6 teaspoons nigari (or other solidifier)
- 2 8–10 quart cooking pots
- 1 blender, food processor, or Corona Mill

- 1 large colander that can sit over the 7–10 quart pot
- 1 1-quart cooking pot
- cheesecloth
- cotton or muslin towel
- spoons, whisk
- large bowl

1. Wash 3 cups yellow soybeans in 9 cups water three times and soak overnight. (For a discussion on the kinds of soybeans to use, see note at the end.)

- Three cups of soybeans (about 19 ounces solid) make about 3 1/2 pounds of tofu (about three times more by weight).
- The soybeans must soak long enough so that the water penetrates all the way to the center of the soybean. To check, split open a soaked soybean. The inside surface of both halves should be flat and white. If the surface is concave, and the middle grayish, the soybeans were not soaked long enough; the yield of tofu will be lower.

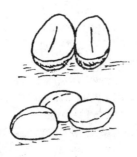

If the soaking water turns sour or the beans break open, they were soaked for too long; the yield of tofu will also be lower.

Soaking may take between 10 hours (in summer) and 20 hours (in winter).

2. Bring 24 cups water to a boil in a 10-quart pot.

3. While the water comes to a boil, drain the soaking wa-

ter of the soybeans and grind to a fine purée:

a) *With a blender or food processor:* set aside 5 cups of the boiling water from the pot and add to the soaked and drained soybeans. Blend 3-4 minutes to make the finest puree possible. Pour into the pot of boiling water, or

b) *With a Corona Mill:* adjust the Corona Mill to the finest setting and grind the soybeans (without water) to make the finest purée possible. When finished, rinse the mill into the pot of boiling water to clean all the small grits of soybeans from the mill, and pour the puréed soybeans into the 24 cups of boiling water.

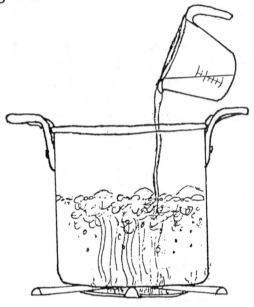

• The finer you grind the soybeans, the more tofu you get. The grounds of soybeans should be about the size of cornmeal. If the beans have been soaked long enough, they are easy to grind very finely.

4. With a whisk, mix the purée and water thoroughly, and heat until it foams. Be careful as the hot liquid foams up suddenly and very quickly, before it comes to a boil. When the foam comes up, lower the flame and sprinkle a few pinch-

es of wheat or rice bran on the foam to bring it down (you may also use sesame oil). It will come up again once or twice; bring it down if necessary.

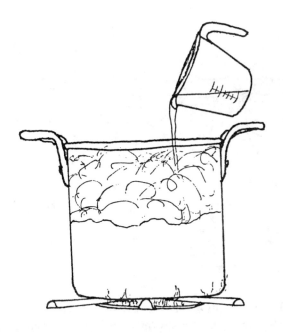

5. Adjust the flame and let simmer gently for 5-15 minutes.
• If the liquid boils too much or for too long (or if it sticks to the bottom of the pot), you will get less tofu. If it does not simmer long enough you will also get less tofu (see discussion on the types of soybeans at the end)

6. Put a colander over another 10-quart pot. Place a coarsely woven cotton towel (muslin, burlap or 5–6 layers of cheesecloth also work well) inside the colander.

7. Pour the boiling liquid through the cloth and colander to filter off the small grits of soybeans (*okara*). Collect the soymilk into a 10-quart pot and keep hot (175 degrees F. is best). You may have to put the pot on a low flame to keep it hot

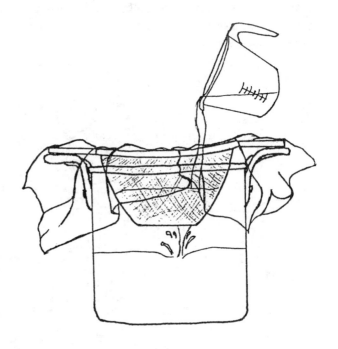

enough.

    • If the cloth you use is woven very coarsely, some okara will go through into the soymilk and the tofu which will be a little gritty: It will make more tofu. If your cloth is woven too fine, it will take a long time to filter and you will get less tofu.

    8. Put 10 cups water into the 10-quart pot you just emptied and bring to a boil.

    9. Using rubber gloves, bring together the corners of the cloth to form a bag, and wring as hard as you can to squeeze all the soymilk out into the pot.

    10. When the 10 cups of water come to a boil, pour the okara from the cloth into the boiling water, lower the flame, and simmer 5 minutes.

    11. Pour the boiling purée through the cloth and colan-

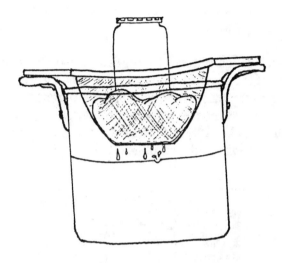

der again (as in #7) and collect the soymilk with the first portion of soymilk already collected in the 10-quart pot.

12. As in #9, extract as much soymilk from the okara as possible.
- The more soymilk you can extract from the okara, the more tofu you get. Also the hotter the okara, the easier it will be to extract more soymilk. You can open the bag, toss the okara and press again for a few minutes using a heavy weight.

13. Remove the colander from over the pot and keep the okara for cooking later (*see below*)
- You should obtain less than 2 pounds of okara. If you have more, you will end up with less tofu. Too much okara means that one of the following is the cause of the problem:
    - The soybeans were not soaked long enough
    - They were not ground fine enough
    - They were under- or overcooked

- The okara has not been pressed enough
- The soybeans are not suited to make tofu

14. While pressing the okara, pour 2 cups water and 6 teaspoons nigari into a small pot. Dissolve the nigari and bring to a boil.
  - Nigari (called bitterns in English) is used to coagulate the proteins of the soymilk to make tofu. When gray sea salt is refined, the gray fraction which contains magnesium chloride, magnesium sulphate, and other minerals is washed off and crystallized: this is nigari. The magnesium ions react with the soybean proteins and coagulates them.

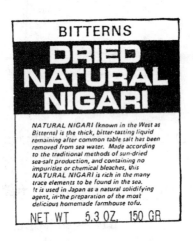

BITTERNS

DRIED NATURAL NIGARI

NATURAL NIGARI (known in the West as Bitterns) is the thick, bitter-tasting liquid remaining after common table salt has been removed from sea water. Made according to the traditional methods of sun-dried sea-salt production, and containing no impurities or chemical bleaches, this NATURAL NIGARI is rich in the many trace elements to be found in the sea. It is used in Japan as a natural solidifying agent, in the preparation of the most delicious homemade farmhouse tofu.

NET WT 5.3 OZ, 150 GR

The amount of nigari needed to coagulate the soymilk can vary widely. Six teaspoons should be a little more than you need for 3 cups of soybeans.
  - If you cannot find nigari you can use food grade Epsom salt (magnesium sulphate) or gypsum (calcium sulphate) which you can find at drug stores. They don't dissolve as easily as nigari. They also make more tofu (but more watery) than nigari. The taste of tofu made with these salts is also inferior to tofu made with nigari.

15. Turn off the flame under the pot of soymilk. If a skin has formed (this is *yuba* and has a delicious taste) on the sur-

face of the milk, remove it.

• The soymilk must be kept hot, but not boiling. If it is not hot enough, much more nigari will be needed to coagulate the soymilk and the tofu will taste bitter and have a hard texture.

16. With a circular motion of a spoon, stir the soymilk a few times to make it spin in the pot. Pour about 1/3 of the nigari liquid into the spinning soymilk. Wait until it stops spinning. With a spoon, sprinkle about 1/3 more nigari liquid on the surface of the soymilk. Put a lid on the pot and let rest 5 minutes.

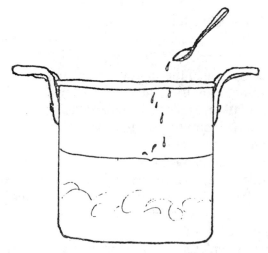

• This is the crucial step. If mixed all at once the nigari and soybean proteins react very quickly making very dense, small curds and hard, crumbly tofu. To make tofu more soft with a nice silky texture, the nigari must be added in 2-3 steps to slow down the coagulation. But if you add the nigari too slowly, say in 4-5 steps, the curds will be very soft and will break easily. They will be difficult to separate from the whey later.

• The curds form into the pot from the bottom up. When you add the nigari it sinks to the bottom, and any soymilk that does not coagulate tends to float on the surface.

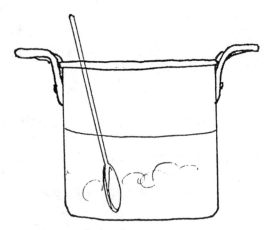

17. Remove the lid. With a spoon, poke the curds gently to dislodge any soymilk that did not coagulate. It should come up to the surface. With a spoon, sprinkle just enough nigari on the surface of the soymilk to coagulate almost all of the remaining soymilk. Gently stir the surface of the milk to assist coagulation. Replace the lid and leave the mixture undisturbed for 15 minutes. Let the curds form completely and settle to the bottom of the pot.

• You must manage to coagulate all the soymilk proteins with as little nigari as possible. If you use more than needed, the tofu will be very firm and crumbly; you will get less tofu. Also, since nigari is very bitter, any excess will give a strong bitter taste to the tofu.

• If you don't use enough nigari, some of the milk will not coagulate; you will get less tofu.

18. While the soymilk coagulates, put the colander over the 10-quart pot and line it with 2 layers of cheesecloth.

19. After 15 minutes the curds should have settled to the bottom of the pot, and there should be a clear yellow liquid above them. This is *whey*. The curds should be about one third of the way down below the surface of the whey. The curds should look somewhat like poached eggs.

• If the whey is very cloudy and white, you need more nigari.

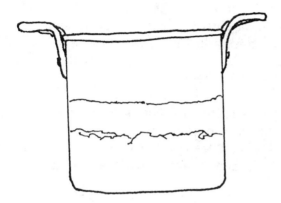

- If it is hazy, you poured the nigari too slowly (or the milk was not hot enough).
- If there is not much curds and the whey is completely clear, you may have added the nigari too quickly, or you did not extract enough protein from the soybeans.

20. First ladle and strain as much whey as possible through the cheesecloth and colander to moisten the cheesecloth thoroughly. Then gently ladle all the curds on the cheesecloth in the colander.

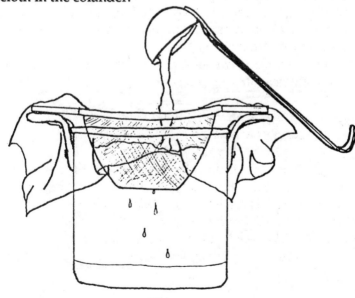

Some whey will remain trapped into the curds. The difference between firm and soft tofu lies in the amount of whey that stays into the curds; the more whey the softer the tofu. If you want soft tofu, ladle the curds very gently to avoid breaking them. If you want firm tofu, lightly break up the curds with a spoon or a rubber spatula.

21. If you wish, you can eat the tofu right away without pressing it. Just let the whey drain and use as it is in soups, sautéed with vegetables, or as an appetizer seasoned with shoyu, scallions, and sesame seeds. That is tofu at its very best.

22. If you want to keep it for later use, you can press it into a solid cake which can be cut into cubes or sliced to boil or pan fry.

Let the tofu rest a few minutes in the colander or the pot, to drain as much whey as possible. Then, gently fold the cheesecloth over to wrap the curds. Put a plate on the curds and a weight on the plate. For soft tofu, put about three pounds weight (which is about 1/2 quart of water into a glass jar).

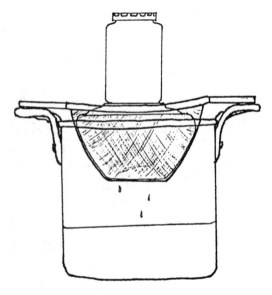

For a firm tofu, put about five pounds weight (about 1 quart of water into a glass jar).

At this stage you can make the tofu a little more or less firm but steps #16–17 and 20 have a much greater influence on the firmness of the tofu.

23. Let the tofu press for about one hour for soft tofu and up to two hours for firm tofu. But be careful. The longer the tofu is left at room temperature, the quicker it will spoil in the refrigerator during the following days.

24. Remove the weight and put the colander and tofu into a large bowl of cold water. Unwrap the tofu and slide it off the cheesecloth and the colander directly into the water. You should obtain about 3-1/2 pounds of tofu depending on the firmness. The more firm, the less tofu.

25. Refrigerate immediately. If you change the soaking water daily, your tofu should keep for one week. You can also store your tofu in a container completely filled with water. Put the lid so that no air remains between the water and the lid. Stored this way, the water does not need to be changed daily.

Soybeans

Not all soybeans can make good tofu. Sometimes, it is difficult to determine if a type of soybean will make a generous quantity of delicious tofu. In general, the bigger, rounder, and sweeter soybeans you can find, the better. There are two great families of soybeans:

• *Vegetable type:* bigger, rounder, sweeter, tastier, more expensive. It is the type grown in Oriental countries to make tofu. Black soybeans are one variety of vegetable soybean. They make wonderful tofu. If you don't remove the skins the tofu will be purple.

• *Field type:* smaller, oval, oily, a bit bitter, cheaper. The type used to make soybean oil in the U.S. is less suited. But some varieties of field soybeans make excellent tofu.

Soybeans that are more than one year old don't yield much tofu. They have to be soaked longer (up to 24 hours). Also when puréed, they have to be cooked longer (step #5), up to 20 minutes.

Make several batches of tofu using the same type of soybeans. If your procedure is correct and you keep getting a low yield, try a different kind.

Okara

If you extract as much liquid as you can from the okara, it will keep very well when refrigerated. Do not put into a tightly closed container; it might turn sour.

Okara is a very rich source of protein and fibers. It has a very nice flavor. You can use it in soups, sautéed with vegetables, or cooked with grains or sea vegetables.

It can be used to make tempeh. The mold that makes tempeh breaks down the proteins of okara and makes it very easy to digest. Okara tempeh has a very light fluffy texture and can be used just like soybean tempeh.

Okara can also be roasted in the oven at 300 degrees F. for 30–60 minutes. It keeps for months this way. You can add it to breads, cookies, or use it instead of nuts as topping for desserts. If you cannot use the okara, you can put it on the compost pile or feed it to animals. It has also been used to polish furniture. You can make a paste with it and rub it into the wood. Let sit and brush the white particles off.

Whey

The whey makes an excellent soap to wash your utensils and pots. It also makes a very nice and mild shampoo (it contains the lecithin of the soybeans).

Soymilk

The procedure for making soymilk is basically the same as for making tofu except for the following:

1. With 3 cups of soybeans you can make 17-23 cups soymilk.

2. Bring either 12 cups water (for thicker soymilk) or 18 cups water (for a thinner soymilk) to a boil in a 10-quart pot..

3. Heat the soaked beans and soaking water to 180 degrees F. Let sit for 15 minutes.
a) Same, but grind hot, or
b) Same but grind hot
Grinding the soybeans hot and pouring immediately in boiling water destroys the enzymes responsible for the beany taste that soymilk might have otherwise.

4. Same

5. Same

6. Same

7. Same

8. Put 4 cups water (for thick or thin soymilk) into the 10-quart pot you just emptied and bring to a boil.

9. Same

10. When the 4 cups water come to a boil, open the cloth, toss the okara, and pour the 4 cups boiling water over it.

11. Omit

12. Same

13. Same

14. Add 3–4 pinches of salt, 3–4 tablespoons of barley malt, and 1 cup of tahini or nut butter if you wish, and simmer 10 minutes.

15. You can drink freshly made; it is delicious. It will keep for one week when refrigerated.

16. If you want to keep it longer, you can sterilize it. Put into mason jars (4 or 5 times 1 quart), cap loosely, and boil 20 minutes. Then screw the caps tightly and store. It will keep for months.

Community Tofu

You can make up to 25 pounds of tofu in about 2 hours. The basic procedure is the same, but there are a few exceptions.

Quantity

In order to make tofu successfully, you must use between 7 and 12 times more water than soybeans (by volume). If you use less, you will not extract enough protein from the soybeans and the soymilk will not coagulate well. You will end up with less tofu than you could. If you use more than 12 times more water, you will need to use much more nigari to coagulate the soymilk. The tofu will be hard and bitter. You will also end up with less tofu than you normally should.

If you wish, you can experiment with different ratios within the margins stated above. If you use less water (say, between 7 and 10 times), you will make less tofu, but it will have a very nice, silky texture and a wonderful taste. If you choose to use more water (between 10 and 12 times), you may make more tofu, but its texture may be more coarse and it may taste bitter.

The following table gives the ratios of ingredients needed to make different quantities of tofu.

Soybeans	Total Water 7–12 times	Maximum Pot Size	Nigari & Water	Okara	Tofu Yield
6 cups	42–72 c.		6 T + 4 c.	4 lb.	5–7 1/2 lb.
10 cups	70–120 c.	10 gal.	7 T + 5 c.	6 lb.	10–12 1/2 lb.
14 cups	98–168 c.	10 gal.	9 T + 7 c.	8 1/2 lb.	14–17 lb.
16 cups	112–192 c.	12 gal.	10 T + 7 c.	9 1/2 lb.	15–20 lb.
20 cups	140-240 c.	15 gal.	12 T + 9 c.	12 lb.	18–24 1/2 lb.
		20 gal.			

Depending on the size of pots you have, the quantity of water may vary. Also the procedure can be modified to accommodate different sizes of pots.

Procedure

a) Equipment

To make large quantities of tofu you will need an electric grinder. A commercial blender or an electric steel burr mill can be used. Grinding soybean does not require much power, but it may take a long time. Choose a grinder that will make the finest puree possible quickly. You will need the biggest stainless steel cooking pots you can find. To cook the soymilk, you may need a portable restaurant gas burner. Choose a strong one. It may take 1/2 hour to bring 10 gallons of soymilk to a boil.

A press for okara can be built with a hydraulic jack on a support. The okara can be wrapped in burlap or coarsely woven nylon sack. The efficiency of the grinder, burner, and the press determines how fast one batch of tofu can be made. With good equipment, 20–25 pounds of tofu can be made in 1 to 2 hours.

b) Procedure

To save time, you may do only one boiling and pressing (steps #2, 3, 4, 5, 7, 9 of homemade procedure) and omit reboiling and repressing (steps #8, 10, 11, 12). That will save about 30 minutes.

But you need to find a bigger cooking pot and a bigger burner. Make sure the cooking pot is not more than 3/4 full when the water and ground soybeans are added. When the milk foams up it needs space to expand without overflowing.

The curdling pot does not have to be a cooking pot. It can be a wooden barrel or any container that will keep the milk hot.

Wooden Pressing Box for Tofu

The curds can be ladled and formed into blocks using a pressing box. This box is very easy to make.

• The wood used must not expand or crack when soaked in water. It must not contain too much acid (tannins) or stains that may stain the tofu. Also, it should have only a light fragrance. Tofu absorbs the odors and tastes of everything it is in contact with. For these reasons the best kinds of wood to use are: cypress, cedar (nonaromatic), mahogany (dark), beech, or maple.

• It is difficult to press thick blocks of tofu. So it is preferable to build shallow boxes that will make blocks of about 3 1/2 to 4 inches thick, no more. During pressing, the volume of curds reduces by about half.

• Since it will stay in water often the box cannot be made using screws that rust. Only brass screws can be used. Also, glue cannot be used. Tofu whey may dissolve it.

• A 1-pound block of tofu measures about 50 cubic inches. The following table gives approximate dimensions for tofu pressing boxes of different sizes.

	height	width	length	thickness wood
2 lb tofu	3 1/2"	3 1/2"	6"	1/2"
10 lb tofu	8"	8"	9"	3/4"
20 lb tofu	9"	9"	14"	3/4"

all inside dimensions

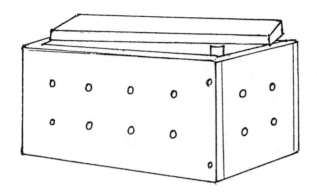

The box can be lined with two long pieces of muslin, one lengthwise, the other widthwise. It is washable and reusable. Cheesecloth can also be used, but it cannot be reused many times.

The base and lid being loose, the box can be dismantled easily under water. After the block of tofu has finished pressing, remove the weight and lid; then slide the box upward. The block of tofu will rest on the base. It can be floated in water to remove the base and unwrap the block of tofu.

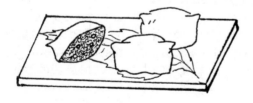

Deep-fried tofu pouches.

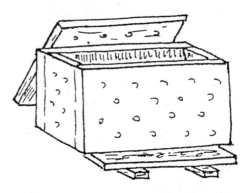

Tofu box: use 3/4-inch-thick wood for 10 pounds of tofu or more.

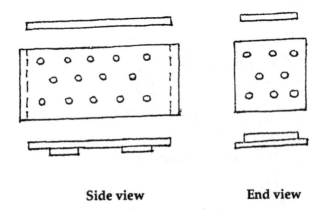

Side view   **End view**

**Cut top and bottom about 1/2-inch smaller than box opening
to allow for expansion of the wood.**

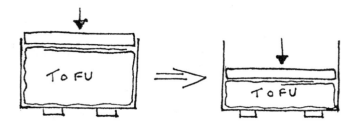

A block of tofu reduces to half of volume of the curds when pressing, so build box accordingly.

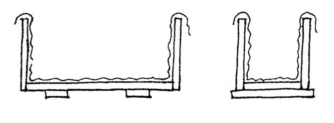

Side view   **End view**

Cloth must overlap sides. Set straight and tight before pressing or it may get trapped in the block of tofu.

Appendix 1

Buying and Storing Grains

Cereal grains and beans can be purchased from natural food stores or from mail order catalogs (*see list below*). Always choose organically grown grains. They usually cost a little more than the commercial varieties, but their quality is much higher. They are grown with care by people who respect the environment and are conscious of the health benefits provided by the foods they grow.

Cereals, like wheat or barley, are harvested in August. Then they are dried for a few weeks and are sold usually at the beginning of September. Rice is harvested later and is usually available fresh at the end of the year. Soybeans are also put on the market around November. During storage, grains and beans lose some water by evaporation and they become harder and more difficult to cook. Try as much as possible to buy grains or beans that are not more than one year old. They often taste "dusty" or stale. Often, they don't sprout; they have lost their vitality. When you make tofu, it is very important to use soybeans that are less than one year old. The yield and the taste of tofu suffers greatly when using old beans.

When buying grains, check carefully the appearance. The number of broken grains, pieces of husks, or foreign materials should be very small (2 to 3 percent). The grains must look "plump," full, not wrinkled. The seed coat or bran must be intact. There should be only a few sparse immature, greenish looking seeds. Check also for moths. They are a constant problem with grains. Their presence is revealed by small clusters of grains bound together by fine threads, clumping to the sides of containers. Also small holes bored through at the center of grains are a sign of infestation. Finally, check for any stale or rancid smell. When you wash grains or beans, they should sink in the water. Any grain that floats is dead. Do not use. There should be only a small fraction of floating grains or chaff. If you find a large quantity, do not use. These grains are old.

Some rice growers (*see list below*) can supply unhulled rice. Rice grows in the field with a hull which protects the grain. Usually, after harvest, the hulls are removed. During shipping and storage, the grains rub against each other and damage the layer of bran. That promotes oxidation of the grains and subsequent loss of nutritive value and freshness. If the hulls are left on the grains, they can keep fresh for much longer, and they don't lose nutritive value. Rice, with the hulls, can keep for years and still sprout.

Millet can also be purchased unhulled. Although barley, spelt, oats, and buckwheat also grow with a hull, they are not usually available as such since they require special equipment to dehull. Wheat and rye do not have hulls.

A small electric rice huller made in Japan is available (*see below*) to hull rice, millet, and to clean grains and beans easily.

Always try to buy flours, cracked grains, and flakes that are as fresh as possible. Flour especially oxidizes very quickly and loses nutritive value and taste within a few weeks. The best flour is freshly ground. If you plan on using flour regularly, investing in a good flour mill is a worthwhile investment (*see below*).

Store grains and beans in a cool, dark, and dry place in containers that shut tightly. Do not store grains on concrete floors or any damp area. Freezing does not disturb grains but heat does. Rotate your stock regularly. Moths make nests only in grains that are left undistrubed for months. If you move your grains from time to time, they will move away.

When you have a problem with infestation, you should thoroughly clean your storage area and put your grains into new containers. Next, put bay leaves in your grains, e.g., 10 to 12 leaves for 50 pounds of grain. That will chase away moths. If your grains are infested with eggs and larvae that have penetrated inside the grains, you can put them in the freezer (or outside in winter) for a few days. That will kill the eggs. Wash these grains very well before using them.

Salt and nigari are very hydroscopic; they absorb moisture very rapidly. And they oxidize metal also. Always store these in a dry place in containers that close tightly. Do not use metallic containers to store them or leave metal utensils in salt or nigari. Wood, glass, or porcelain are the best materials used to handle salt.

Equipment

I do most of the food processing by hand. Having worked in many different food factories equipped with very sophisticated machinery, I highly value the quiet and silent manual work. When I need a piece of equipment to facilitate my work, I am very selective. I manage to keep it to a minimum. I choose equipment that I can repair and control easily. I avoid machines that impose their mechanical rhythm on me. If possible, I build them. Most of the equipment needed can be built fairly easily.

Some others must be purchased. Following is a description of a few pieces that are very useful to transform grains and beans. They are multi-purpose and easy to use. They are available from many suppliers (*see list below*) by mail order.

Rice Huller

At the Kushi Institute we have a small electric huller from Japan. It can hull rice, sweet rice, buckwheat, and millet. It can clean grains and beans. When I make tempeh, I separate the hulls of soybeans from the beans with it. I also use it to

**Rice Hulling
Machine**

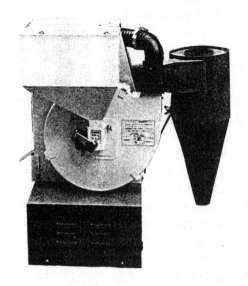

remove the rootlets and husks of malted barley. It measures 23 x 10 x 23 inches. It is very easy to use. You just pour the un-hulled rice into the hopper, turn the machine on, and open the small auger trap. The hulled rice comes out from one end of the machine and the hulls are blown out through a cyclone into a bag. It can hull 100 pounds of rice per hour. It can be adjusted to hull different grains. We have been using this machine in Becket to hull our rice for many years. We use about 15 pounds of rice per day. It never fails and is very simple to maintain.

If you want to experiment, there are other ways to hull rice. It is very easy to hull. In the past, people used a large mortar and pestle to hull rice and a flail to separate the hulls from the grains. But a few grains are broken in the process. I have heard about someone using a Corona Mill (*see below*) to hull rice. He removes the steel burrs from the mill and replaces them with discs of thick rubber of the same diameter as the original metal plates. Some rice growers hull their rice by using a machine whose main parts are two rubber cylinders which turn at different speeds (a little bit like the old style clothes wringer of your grandmother's washing machine). The hulls of the rice pop off as it passes between the cylinders. The distance between these two must be adjusted precisely to avoid breaking the grains.

Steel Plates Mill

One piece of equipment that is very useful is a manual steel mill. Two companies manufacture them. One is called a Corona Mill, the other a Quaker Mill. The Corona mill is a very inexpensive corn mill made in Colombia (where corn is a staple). It is very easy to use and very strong. I have been using one for years to grind soaked soybeans to make tofu, mochi, corn masa, sprouted wheat bread, and more. I also use it to crack soybeans to make tempeh. The manufacturer offers a "stone conversion bit," which is a pair of stones (synthetic) used to make flour. The steel burrs will grind humid grains or cracked grains easily, but they cannot make flour. I did not use their "stone conversion bit." To make flour, it is preferable to buy a good flour mill.

Although the manufacturer does not recommend it, I motorized my Corona Mill. I used a 1/4 H.P. electric motor and reduced the speed (motor 1725 R.P.M.) to 100 R.P.M. of the mill with a combination of pulleys and belts. Since this mill is made of soft steel and has no bearings, I made sure it turned slowly enough to prevent excessive wear of the metal. The slower speed also increases the available power of the motor. I keep the shaft of the mill oiled with a little bit of cooking oil. At that speed, it grinds 6 pounds of soybeans (for making tofu) in 10 minutes.

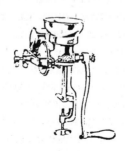

Flour Mill

To grind flour properly, you need a stone mill. These may be either manual or electric. If you use 3 to 4 cups or less of flour at a time, a manual mill is adequate. But if you make more, an electric mill would often be more useful.

There are many different kinds of manual mills available, and they all do more or less a good job. There is one that is worth mentioning: the Samap manual flour mill. It is very well made, not too strenuous to use, and can make very fine flour rapidly.

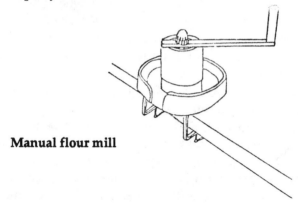

Manual flour mill

Electric mills also are made by many different manufacturers. They can make between 5 and 100 pounds of flour per hour. Choose a mill that grinds flour more slowly. If the mill turns too fast, it heats the flour and destroys some of the nutritive value of the grain. The flour should come out from between the stones slightly warm (100 to 110 degrees F.), not hot. This is especially important if you make naturally leavened bread. You must not destroy the enzymes and microorganisms of the wheat during milling.

In Becket, I use two stone mills. One is smaller. It is a Mil-Rite flour mill built by Retsel. It is built very simply: a motor, two stones, and a hopper. The stones turn very slowly: only 60 R.P.M. So the flour never heats up. It can grind four cups (the capacity of the hopper) of wheat in about 10 minutes. It comes with a detachable handle that allows you to

Mill Rite
flour mill

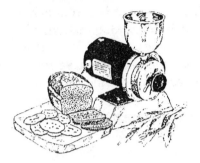

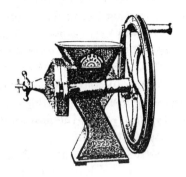

D525 Diamant
flour mill

grind flour manually if you do not want to use the motor. It can grind wheat, rice, barley, rye, buckwheat, and corn. The stones are infinitely adjustable to grind coarse up to very fine flour. It is built very strong and heavy. It does not need to be bolted to a table and is not messy. Some mills are cumbersome to use and difficult to clean. This one very seldom needs to be disassembled. It sells for about $250. I use it to grind the flour to make the leaven and for small needs.

The second mill I use is a Diamant type D-525 made in Denmark. It is made of cast iron, very heavy, and needs to be bolted securely to a heavy table. It comes equipped with a large pulley that can be coupled to a 1/2 H.P. motor. A handle (removable) screwed to the rim of the pulley allows you to grind flour manually if you wish. The grain is fed to the grinding plate by a long screw with teeth that crack the grains before they reach the plates. That greatly facilitates the grinding. It comes with three sets of metal grinding plates (removable) with grooves of different depths that can be used to make flakes, coarse and fine grits, or flour. A pair of stones can also be installed on this mill to make very fine wheat flour. The distance between the plates can be adjusted easily to make any kind of grind desired. The hopper can hold 7 cups of grains. It can mill (when motor-powered) about 40 pounds of flour or 110 pounds of cracked grains per hour. By hand, it can make about 10 pounds of flour per hour. Since the pulley is large, it can be turned fairly easily. It takes a bit longer to disassemble than the Mil Rite mill when it needs cleaning, but not excessively so. It sells for approximately $350 with metal plates, plus $25 per set of extra steel plates and $50 for a set of stones. I have used this mill for years to make bread, seitan, pastries, soy sauce (to crack the wheat), and more. And it has always been very reliable.

In the past, the flour mills were equipped with natural stones (sandstone or granite). But today, the stones are made of particles of granite embedded in a very strong cement. They very seldom wear out and never need to be redressed and sharpened. In the old mills, the stones had to be re-dressed about once per month. There is only one manufacturer in the United States that still uses natural granite stones: Meadow Mill. They make probably the best flour mill in this country. But their smaller model is a little bit too big for home use.

Although the new types of stones are, in general, reliable, they are not equal. Some stones will chip more easily and particles of stone dust may end up in your flour. They will wear out faster and may break. These stones cannot be redressed. So check carefully before buying a stone mill.

Making Flour

The grains you use must be dry enough to be ground into flour. If they are too humid, they will clog the grooves of the plates or the stones, covering them with a hard shiny coat that makes grinding impossible. If your grains are too humid, you can put them in the oven at 250 degrees F. for 30 to 60 minutes before grinding.

Stone mills cannot be used to grind wet or oily grains or seeds, only cereal grains. Metal plate mills are used preferably for nuts, soybeans, or wet ingredients. They can also be used to grind flour, but since they cannot grind as finely as stones, they must be adjusted at a very fine setting to grind flour fine enough. In consequence, the flour is heated much more than when using stones. The very fine particles on the surface of the stones can very finely grind the hardest grain. Wheat is the most difficult grain to grind into flour because it is very hard. Also since the surface of the stones can grind more easily than metal plates, the stone mills can achieve their purpose by turning at a lower speed than metal mills. They don't overheat flour.

White Flour

If you want to sift your flour to obtain white flour, you must grind your wheat in a special way. You must increase the moisture of the wheat berries before grinding them. When the grain is dry, the bran is very brittle and is pulverized between the stones during milling. If you increase the moisture slightly, the grain becomes more flexible and slides between the stones . It comes out in large pieces which can be separated from the flour easily. You need to increase the moisture of the wheat berries from 13 percent (when you buy it) to 18 to 20 percent or thereabouts. To 10 pounds of wheat berries, add 1 1/2 cups of water and mix thoroughly. Let sit overnight. Mix from time to time. Then grind. Do not use too much water. If the grain is too humid, it will clog the stones and make a mess. You will have to dismantle the mill and clean the stones.

Bulgur

Bulgur is very simple to make. The next time you want some, instead of buying it, make it yourself. Here is how. Choose a variety of wheat that is very hard and vitreous. To test, bite one grain and check the interior: it must have a glassy luster. Varieties of wheat that have a starchy interior will not work very well. Sometimes durum wheat is used to make bulgur. Wash it and soak it overnight. The next day, boil in about 2 times as much water and a little bit of salt until cooked, but still firm, about 1 hour. When done, drain well, spread on a baking sheet, and dry in the oven at 250 to 300 degrees F. until it becomes hard. Do not roast the grains. Stir from time to time, grind coarsely, and store. It will keep for months.

Buckwheat Flour

In my hometown, there is a flour mill that was built in the seventeenth century by French settlers in Quebec. It is still running today with the original waterwheel, the enormous wooden gears, and the original stones. The two sets of stones still grind very fine wheat and buckwheat flour today for the enjoyment of the neighborhood.

The buckwheat flour produced at this mill is the best I have ever seen, very light, soft, and white. (It makes the best buckwheat pancakes.) One day, I went to visit the miller and asked him how he did such flour. He told me that the two sets of stones were different: one was for wheat, the other one for buckwheat. He uses a very sharp and heavy stone to grind wheat flour for some years. Then when it wears out, he uses it to grind buckwheat flour. When the grains of buckwheat pass between the dull stones, the husks slide between the stones and come out in big pieces that are very easy to separate from the flour. Today, buckwheat flour is usually made either with a metal burrs or a hammer mill. These pulverize the husks which end up in the flour. The flour produced by the buckwheat grains is very white and light; it is very easy to grind finely. But it is the presence of husks that makes the flour black and heavy.

One way to make good buckwheat flour for soba noodles is to coarsely grind unhulled buckwheat kernels in a stone mill, then sift. You may have to grind the flour a second time to make it fine enough. If you have the opportunity, try it. You will be surprised to see how soft and delicate buckwheat can be.

Cooking Utensils

Large stainless steel pots, bowls, and pans are available at restaurant suppliers and commercial kitchen suppliers, as well as equipment like commercial sized blenders, gas burners, and grinders that can be very useful. Check also at amateur beer and wine makers' stores. They carry barrels, wine presses, strainers, tubes, thermometers, and many other pieces of equipment that can be used to make natural foods.

There is only one manufacturer of large pressure cookers that I know of. It is Wisconsin Aluminum Foundries. They make cast aluminum pressure cookers. They make many different sizes, from 7 quarts to 41 1/2 quarts. You can cook about 25 pounds of rice with the larger cooker. Their prices range from $125 to $250 apiece.

Suppliers

Gold Mine Natural Foods
1947 30th St.
San Diego, CA 92102
619-234-9711

Natural Lifestyle Supplies
16 Lookout Drive
Asheville, NC 28804
800-752-2775

Albion Enterprises (cookware)
3233 Coffey Lane, Suite H
Santa Rosa, CA 95403

R&R Mill (Corona Mills, etc.)
45 West First North
Smithfield, UT 84335
801-563-3333

Wisconsin Aluminum Foundry (large pressure cookers)
P.O. Box 246
Manitowoc, WI 54221-0246

Miracle Exclusives (flour mills)
P.O. Box 349
Locust Valley, NY 11560

Diamant Domestic Grain Mills
Box 123
D.V. Station
Dayton, OH 45406

Mountain Ark Trading Co.
120 S. East St.
Fayetteville, AR 72701
800-643-8909

Lundberg Farms (unhulled rice)
5370 Church St.
P.O. Box 369
Richvale, CA 95974

Southern Brown Rice (rice)
P.O. Box 185
Weiner, AR 72479
501-684-2354

G.E.M. Cultures (koji, starters)
30301 Sherwood Rd.
Fort Bragg, CA 95437

Lehman's Catalog
P.O. Box 41
4779 Kidron Rd.
Kidron, OH 44636

Macrobiotic Wholesale Co. (bulk grains and beans)
799 Old Leicester Highway
Asheville, NC 28806
800-438-4730

Measures

1 tablespoon salt = 25.30 grams (about 1 ounce)
1 cup salt = 8 ounces (solid)
1 cup soybeans = 6.5 ounces (solid)
1 quart soybeans = 1.65 pounds
1 cup rice = 7 ounces (solid)
1 cup wheat = 7 ounces (solid)
1 cup flour = 6 ounces (solid)
1 cup water = 6 ounces (solid)
1 gallon water = 8.3 pounds

Grains and Beans Preparation
rice: 1 pound raw gives 1.40 pounds soaked
sweet rice: 1 pound raw gives 1.35 pounds soaked
soybeans: 1 pound raw gives 2.2 pounds soaked with
    60 percent moisture

Raw grains and beans when purchased usually
    contain 13 to 15 percent moisture

Salt should not contain more than 5 percent moisture

3 teaspoons = 1 tablespoon = 1/2 fluid ounce
16 tablespoons = 1 cup = 8 fluid ounces
2 cups = 1 pint = 16 fluid ounces
4 cups = 1 quart = 32 fluid ounces
4 quarts = 1 gallon = 128 fluid ounces

1 ounces = 28.3 grams
1 pound = 453.6 grams
1 tablespoon = 14.7 milligrams

1 fluid ounce = 29.6 milligrams
1 cup = 236 milligrams
1 quart = 0.946 liter
1 gallon (U.S.) = 3.785 liters

temperature C. = 5/9 (F. -32)
temperature F. = (1.8 x C.) + 32
boiling water = 212° F. = 100° C.
freezing water = 32° F. = 0° C.
body temperature = 98.6° F. = 37° C.

Appendix 2

Standard Macrobiotic Dietary Guidelines*

Foods for Daily Consumption

• **Whole Cereal Grains:** The principal food of each meal is whole cereal grain, comprising from 50 to 60 percent of the total volume. Whole grains include brown rice, whole wheat berries, barley, millet, and rye, as well as corn, buckwheat, and other botanically similar plants. From time to time, whole grain products, such as cracked wheat, rolled oats, noodles, pasta, bread, baked goods, and other unrefined flour products, may be served as part of this volume.

• **Soup:** One to two small bowls of soup, making up about 5 to 10 percent of daily food intake, are consumed each day. The soup broth is made frequently with miso or shoyu and also includes vegetable, bean, and grain soups.

• **Vegetables:** About 25 to 30 percent of daily food includes fresh vegetables prepared in a variety of ways, including steaming, boiling, baking, sautéing, salads, and marinades. The vegetables include a variety of root vegetables (such as cabbage, carrots, and daikon radish), ground vegetables (such as onions and fall-and winter-season squashes), and leafy green vegetables (such as kale, collard greens, broccoli, turnip greens, mustard greens, and watercress).

• **Beans and Sea Vegetables:** A small portion, about 10 percent by volume, of daily food intake includes cooked beans such as adukis, lentils, and chickpeas or bean products such as tofu, tempeh, and natto and sea vegetables, including kombu, wakame, nori, dulse, hijiki, and arame.

• **Seasoning and Oil:** Naturally processed sea salt is used in seasoning, along with miso, shoyu, umeboshi, brown rice vinegar, fresh grated ginger and other traditional items. Naturally processed, unrefined vegetable oil is recommended for daily cooking such as dark sesame seed oil. Kuzu is commonly used for gravies and sauces.

• **Condiments:** Condiments include gomashio (roasted sesame salt), roasted seaweed powders, umeboshi plums, tekka root vegetables, and many others.

• **Pickles:** A small volume of home-made pickles is eaten each day to aid in digestion of grains and vegetables.

• **Beverages:** Spring or well water is used for drinking, preparing tea, and for general cooking. Bancha twig tea (also known as kukicha) is the most commonly served beverage, though roasted barley tea, and other grain-based teas or traditional, nonstimulant herbal teas are also used frequently.

Occasional Foods for Those in Usual Good Health

• **Animal Food:** A small volume of white-meat fish or seafood may be eaten a few times per week.

• **Seeds and Nuts:** Seeds and nuts, lightly roasted and salted with sea salt or seasoned with shoyu, may be enjoyed as occasional snacks.

• **Fruit:** Fruit may be taken a few times a week, preferably cooked or naturally dried, as a snack or dessert, provided the fruit grows in the local or similar climate zone.

• **Dessert:** Occasional desserts may consist of cookies, pudding, cake, pie, and other dishes made with naturally sweet foods such as apples, fall- and winter-season squashes, aduki beans, or dried fruit or may be sweetened with a natural grain-based sweetener such as amasake, barley malt, or rice syrup.

These guidelines are for four-season temperate climates including most of the United States and Canada, Europe, Russia, and China. For guidelines for tropical, semitropical, polar, and semipolar climates, please see Michio Kushi, Standard Macrobiotic Diet (One Peaceful World Press, 1991).

Way of Life Suggestions

• Live each day happily without being preoccupied with your health; try to keep mentally and physically active.

• View everything and everyone you meet with gratitude, particularly offering thanks before and after every meal.

• Please chew your food very well, at least 50 times per mouthful, or until it becomes liquid.

• It is best to avoid wearing synthetic or woolen clothes directly on the skin. As much as possible, wear cotton, especially for undergarments. Avoid excessive metallic accessories on the fingers, wrists, or neck. Keep such ornaments simple and graceful.

• If your strength permits, go outdoors in simple clothing. Walk on the grass, beach, or soil up to one-half hour every day. Keep your home in good order, from the kitchen, bathroom, bedroom, and living rooms, to every corner of the house.

• Initiate and maintain an active correspondence, extending your best wishes to parents, children, brothers and sisters, teachers, and friends.

• Avoid taking long hot baths or showers unless you have been consuming too much salt or animal food.

• To increase circulation, scrub your entire body with a hot, damp towel every morning or every night. If that is not possible, at least scrub your hands, feet, fingers, and toes.

- Avoid chemically perfumed cosmetics. For care of the teeth, brush with natural preparations or sea salt.

- If your condition permits, exercise regularly as part of daily life, including activities like walking, scrubbing floors, cleaning windows, washing clothes and working in the garden. You may also participate in exercise programs such as yoga, martial arts, dance, or sports.

- Avoid using electric cooking devices (ovens and ranges) or microwave ovens. Convert to gas or wood-stove cooking at the earliest opportunity.

- It is best to minimize the use of color television and computer display units.

- Include some large green plants in your house to freshen and enrich the oxygen content of the air of your home.

- Sing a happy song each day.

Resources

One Peaceful World

One Peaceful World is an international information network and friendship society founded by Michio and Aveline Kushi. Its members include individuals, families, educational centers, organic farmers, teachers, parents and children, authors and artists, homemakers and business people, and others devoted to the realization of one healthy, peaceful world. Activities include educational and spiritual tours, assemblies and forums, international food aid and environmental awareness, One Peaceful World Press, and other activities to help humanity pass safely into a new world of planetary health and peace.

Annual membership is $30 for individuals, $50 for families, and $100 for supporting members. Benefits include the quarterly *One Peaceful World Newsletter*, discounts of selected books, cassettes, and videos, and special mailings and communications.

To enroll or for further information, contact:

One Peaceful World
Box 10
Becket, MA 01223
(413) 623–2322
Fax (413) 623–8827

Kushi Institute

A center for macrobiotic and holistic studies located in the Berkshire mountains of western Massachusetts offering year-round programs and seminars in macrobiotic cooking, Far Eastern philosophy and medicine, natural foods processing, spiritual development training, and other disciplines. For further information, please contact:

Kushi Institute
Box 7
Becket, MA 01223
(413) 623–5741
Fax (413) 623–8827

Kushi Foundation Store

The Kushi Foundation Store in Becket carries a mail-order selection of cookware, books, and natural foods, including some bulk items. Information is also available for purchasing the rice hulling machine.

Kushi Foundation Store
Box 7
Becket, MA 01223
(413) 623-2102

Recommended Reading

Books

1. *The Book of Macrobiotics*. Michio Kushi with Alex Jack. Japan Publications, 1986, paperback, $15.95.
2. *One Peaceful World*. Michio Kushi with Alex Jack. St. Martin's Press, 1987, hardcover, $17.95.
3. *Other Dimensions: Exploring the Unexplained*. Michio Kushi with Edward Esko. Avery Publishing Group, 1991, paperback, $9.95.
4. *Food Governs Your Destiny*. Michio and Aveline Kushi, with Alex Jack. Japan Publications, 1991, paperback, $12.95.
5. *The Cancer-Prevention Diet*. Michio Kushi with Alex Jack. St. Martin's Press; revised, expanded, and updated edition, 1993; hardcover, price forthcoming.
6. *Diet for a Strong Heart*. Michio Kushi with Alex Jack. St. Martin's Press, 1985, paperback, $10.95.
7. *The Book of Do In*. Michio Kushi. Japan Publications, 1979, paperback, $14.95.
8. *Cancer-Free: 30 Who Triumphed Over Cancer Naturally*. East West Foundation, with Ann Fawcett and Cynthia Smith. Japan Publications, 1992, paperback, $15.95.
9. *Recovery: From Cancer to Health through Macrobiotics*. Elaine Nussbaum. Avery Publishing Group, 1993, paperback, $9.95.
10. *Macrobiotics and Oriental Medicine*. Michio Kushi

with Phillip Jannetta. Japan Publications, 1991, paperback, $18.95.

11. *Natural Healing through Macrobiotics*. Michio Kushi, with Edward Esko and Marc Van Cauwenberghe, M.D. Japan Publications, 1979, paperback, $14.95.

12. *The Macrobiotic Approach to Cancer*. Michio Kushi, with Edward Esko. Avery Publishing Group, 1991, paperback, $9.95.

13. *Macrobiotic Home Remedies*. Michio Kushi, with Marc Van Cauwenberghe, M.D. Japan Publications, 1985, paperback, $15.95.

14. *Macrobiotic Diet*. Micho and Aveline Kushi, with Alex Jack. Japan Publications, 1993, paperback, $17.00.

15. *AIDS, Macrobiotics, and Natural Immunity*. Michio Kushi, with Martha Cottrell, M.D. Japan Publications, 1990, paperback, $19.95.

16. *Standard Macrobiotic Diet*. Michio Kushi. One Peaceful World Press, 1991, paperback, $5.95.

17. *Nine Star Ki*. Michio Kushi, with Edward Esko. One Peaceful World Press, 1991, paperback, $12.95.

18. *Let Food Be Thy Medicine*. Alex Jack. One Peaceful World Press, 1991, paperback, $10.95.

19. *Macrobiotic Palm Healing*. Michio Kushi, with Olivia Oredson. Japan Publications, 1989, paperback, $15.95.

20. *Promenade Home: Macrobiotics and Women's Health*. Gale and Alex Jack. Japan Publications, 1988, paperback, $18.95.

21. *How to See Your Health*. Michio Kushi. Japan Publications, 1980, paperback, $12.95.

22. *Your Face Never Lies*. Michio Kushi. Avery Publishing Group, 1983, paperback, $9.95.

23. *Healing Planet Earth*. Edward Esko, One Peaceful World Press, 1992, paperback, $5.95.

24. *Notes from the Boundless Frontier*. Edward Esko, One Peaceful World Press, 1992, paperback, $5.95.

25. *Amber Waves of Grain: American Macrobiotic Cooking*. Alex and Gale Jack, Japan Publications, 1992, paperback, $17.00.

26. *Out of Thin Air: A Satire About Owls and Ozone, Beef and Biodiversity, Grains and Global Warming.* Alex Jack, One Peaceful World Press, 1993, paperback, $7.95.

27. *The Teachings of Michio Kushi.* Michio Kushi, edited by Edward Esko, One Peaceful World Press, 1993, paperback, $12.95.

Publications

One Peaceful World, Becket, Massachusetts
MacroNews, Philadelphia, Pennsylvania
Macrobiotics Today, Oroville, California

Books by Mail Order

The books listed above are available by mail-order from One Peaceful World Press. Please make check or money order payable to One Peaceful World and enclose shipping and handling of $1.75 for the first book and .75 for each additional book.

Outside U.S., please pay in U.S. funds drawn on a U.S. bank and enclose 20% of total order for surface mail and 40% for airmail.

Visa or Mastercard also accepted in payment. Please enclose card number, expiration date, and authorized signature.

About the Author

Guy Lalumiere grew up in Canada. In the mid-'70s, a friend introduced him to macrobiotics, and he quit his studies in biochemistry to work in natural food stores in Montreal and study traditional philosophy and medicine. He has been studying with Michio and Aveline Kushi since the mid-'80s.

In 1989, he traveled to the Far East and served as an apprentice in making miso and shoyu at traditional factories in Japan. Since his return, he has taught natural foods processing throughout North America.